CEREBRAL VENOUS THROMBOSIS

Volume 33 in the Series

Major Problems in Neurology
PROFESSOR CP WARLOW, BA, MB, BChir, MD, FRCP
PROFESSOR J VAN GIJN, MD, FRCPE
Consulting Editors

OTHER MONOGRAPHS IN THE SERIES

Barnett, Foster and Hudgson: **Syringomyelia**
Dubowitz and Brooke: **Muscle Biopsy: A Modern Approach**
Pallis and Lewis: **The Neurology of Gastrointestinal Disease**
Hutchinson and Acheson: **Strokes**
Gubbay: **The Clumsy Child**
Hankinson and Banna: **Pituitary and Parapituitary Tumours**
Behan and Currie: **Clinical Neuroimmunology**
Cartlidge and Shaw: **Head Injury**
Lisak and Barchi: **Myasthenia Gravis**
Johnson, Lambie and Spalding: **Neurocardiology: The Interrelationship between Dysfunction in the Nervous and Cardiovascular Systems**
Parkes: **Sleep and its Disorders**
Hopkins: **Headache Problems in Diagnosis and Management**
Wood and Anderson: **Neurological Infections**
Critchley: **Neurological Emergencies**
Ross: **Syncope**
Donaldson: **Neurology and Pregnancy** SECOND EDITION
Porter: **Epilepsy: 100 Elementary Principles** SECOND EDITION
Harper: **Myotonic Dystrophy** SECOND EDITION
Harper: **Huntington's Disease**
Sjaastad: **Cluster Headache Syndrome**
Hodges: **Transient Amnesia: Clinical and Neuropsychological Aspects**
Vermeulen, Lindsay and Van Gijn: **Subarachnoid Haemorrhage**
Bauer and Hanefeld: **Multiple Sclerosis**
Hankey and Warlow: **Transient Ischaemic Attacks of the Brain and Eye**
Zakrzewska: **Trigeminal Neuralgia**
Hilton-Jones, Squier, Taylor and Matthews: **Metabolic Myopathies**
Harper: **Huntington's Disease** SECOND EDITION
Acheson and Saunders: **Neurophthalmology**

CEREBRAL VENOUS THROMBOSIS

MARIE-GERMAINE BOUSSER
Head of the Department of Neurology
Sainte-Antoine Hospital and
Professor of Neurology
Paris VI University, France

and

RALPH ROSS RUSSELL
Honorary Consultant Physician to the National Hospital for Neurology and Neurosurgery,
St Thomas' Hospital and Moorfields Eye Hospital
London, UK

W. B. Saunders Company Ltd
London · Philadelphia · Toronto · Sydney · Tokyo

W. B. Saunders Company Ltd 24–28 Oval Road
London NW1 7DX, UK

The Curtis Center
Independence Square West
Philadelphia, PA 19106–3399, USA

Harcourt Brace & Company
55 Horner Avenue
Toronto, Ontario M8Z 4X6, Canada

Harcourt Brace & Company, Australia
30–52 Smidmore Street
Marrickville, NSW 2204, Australia

Harcourt Brace & Company, Japan
Ichibancho Central Building, 22–1 Ichibancho
Chiyoda-ku, Tokyo 102, Japan

This book is printed on acid-free paper

A catalogue record for this book is available from the British Library

ISBN 0–7020–1937–2

Typeset by Phoenix Photosetting, Chatham, Kent
Printed and bound in Great Britain by The University Press, Cambridge

Contents

To Flora and to Patrick

Series Editor's Foreword

Marie-Germaine Bousser and Ralph Ross Russell have already written extensively on intracranial venous thrombosis in various original papers and now they have put their expertise together in a book to cover the whole subject.

Look in a general medical or neurology textbook and you are likely to find references to intracranial venous thrombosis in one or more places but to find all of them, you will have to search the index under various headings. Cortical venous thrombosis will be found in sections on coma and encephalopathy; dural sinus thrombosis in sections on headache or raised intracranial pressure; and there will probably be something somewhere in the chapter on stroke. This is because intracranial venous thrombosis has a number of different causes and, in itself, is not really a diagnosis because when it is demonstrated the question is immediately: 'why has this particular patient occluded his intracranial veins at this particular time?' Furthermore, a patient may present to an ophthalmologist with transient obscurations of vision, to a neurologist with headache, to a neurosurgeon with possible subarachnoid haemorrhage and even to an infectious diseases specialist with apparent encephalitis. It is an easy diagnosis to miss because unless you think of it, you will not see the subtle changes on an unenhanced CT brain scan and you will not ask for the appropriate imaging of the intracranial veins. Anyway, what is the most appropriate imaging strategy in these days of rapidly advancing MR technology? And how can intracranial venous thrombosis be diagnosed early and treated effectively?

For all these reasons it is a pleasure to introduce a monograph on the subject written by two neurologists who are both extremely well known in the cerebrovascular field. Marie-Germaine Bousser and Ralph Ross Russell are also general neurologists, which is important because intracranial venous thrombosis presents more often to a general neurology service than to a specialised stroke service.

This book emphasises the importance of early diagnosis and early treatment. It provides practical guidance for neurologists and at the same time will give researchers a starting point from which they can develop our still rather rudimentary knowledge of this relatively uncommon but nonetheless important condition.

Charles Warlow,
Edinburgh, September 1996

Introduction

The last two decades have seen a burgeoning interest in the cerebral circulation and in cerebral vascular disease. However, this has been almost exclusively in the behaviour of cerebral arteries, and in the causes of arterial occlusion and rupture. The role of venous obstruction has been largely ignored or forgotten. This book is an attempt to redress the balance and to put venous disease of the brain into its proper perspective.

The reasons for this neglect are easy to understand: cerebral venous thrombosis is a relatively rare condition, until recently it has been difficult to diagnose and, even when it has been demonstrated, the significance of venous thrombosis has been in some doubt.

Estimates of the frequency of cerebral venous disease vary widely and early reports were based purely on findings at autopsy. Figures from the Registrar General of England and Wales (population approximately 56 million) from 1952 to 1961 quote an annual incidence of only 21.7 cases (Kalbag and Woolf, 1967) and a mere 29 cases were discovered in an autopsy survey from Toronto, Canada covering 20 years (Barnett and Hyland, 1953). This contrasts with a prevalence figure of 9% found in 182 consecutive autopsies by Towbin in 1973 and rates of one per 1666–3000 pregnancies quoted by Carroll *et al.* (1966), and an even higher figure by Srinivasan (1983).

These discrepancies are caused by differences in case ascertainment, reflecting the difficulties of diagnosis during life. There is little doubt that most reports in the past have greatly underestimated the frequency of the condition.

In spite of increasing awareness, cerebral venous thrombosis is still a disease in which the correct diagnosis is frequently overlooked or delayed. This is because of the wide spectrum of clinical presentations both in terms of the speed of onset and the range of symptoms. These may include headache, epileptic seizures, altered consciousness and focal cerebral deficits, either transient of permanent. The occurrence of these symptoms, separately or together, should always raise the possibility of venous thrombosis, although the differential diagnosis embraces a wide variety of conditions such as migraine, transient ischaemic attacks, subarachnoid haemorrhage, encephalitis, cerebral abscess and hypertensive encephalopathy. Furthermore, cerebral venous thrombosis often occurs as a complication of pregnancy, of a systemic disease or as a side effect of treatment. As such it can present a diagnostic problem not only to neurologists but to obstetricians, haematologists, oncologists and specialists in infectious disease. Further examples of the diversity of the clinical symptomatology are found in Chapter 3.

The greatly increased diagnostic precision afforded by angiography and more recently by magnetic resonance imaging has enabled partial or complete thrombosis of the cerebral veins and sinuses to be recognized with increasing ease and frequency, and the range of underlying causes has also expanded rapidly. In the last century local infections, mainly otitic, often combined with dehydration, accounted for the majority of cases of sinus thrombosis, whereas infective causes of this kind are now relatively rare. At the present time, even with the most sophisticated haematological laboratory techniques, no abnormality can be found in about one quarter of cases. In spite of this, there is much current interest in the new prothrombotic states, acquired or congenital, occurring with haematological disease or in association with systemic disorders. Pregnancy and the puerperium remain important antecedents of cerebral venous thrombosis, although the underlying abnormality remains largely unexplained.

Pathologists in the last century were familiar with thrombosis in cerebral veins or sinuses found during routine autopsies, but the significance of the finding was sometimes in doubt. The patients had often died from cachexia, malignant disease or cardiac failure, and in many cases no cerebral symptoms had been noticed during life. Sometimes venous thrombosis was associated with regions of brain swelling, infarction or haemorrhage but on other occasions no such abnormalities were present. It was assumed, probably correctly, that in these cases cerebral venous thrombosis was a terminal event of little clinical significance. On the other hand early pathologists were well aware of cerebral infarction and haemorrhage associated with occlusion of the superficial veins or sinuses, and also appreciated the importance of propagation of thrombus from veins to sinuses or vice versa.

The anatomy of the superficial and deep venous systems of the brain is summarized in Chapter 1. There is little to add to older descriptions of morphology but clinical studies have emphasized the importance of anastomotic veins on the cerebral surface and within the substance of the brain, and the role that these may play after vein occlusion as alternative channels of venous drainage. These collateral veins may enlarge considerably during this process and come to resemble venous or arterio-venous malformations, lesions previously thought to be of congenital origin. The unique part played by the arachnoid villi of the superior sagittal sinus in the circulation of cerebrospinal fluid makes intracranial hypertension a cardinal feature of venous thrombosis at this site. Symonds pointed out many years ago that this could occur in the absence of other features of venous infarction and it now appears that the sinus need not be completely occluded and that partial occlusion or even a state of sustained venous hypertension may be sufficient to cause an abnormal rise in cerebrospinal fluid pressure. It now seems likely that impaired venous drainage may be responsible for some cases previously thought of as 'benign intracranial hypertension'.

The under-recognition of cerebral venous disease would be of little practical importance were it not for the fact that prognosis, management and treatment are very different from that on the arterial side of the circulation, and that these differences are not widely known. The potential for recovery in cerebral venous thrombosis is much greater than that after arterial occlusion. Even patients in coma with dense focal signs persisting for days or weeks may show a remarkable improvement. Furthermore it now appears very probable that as a result of the important trial conducted by Einhäupl and his group in Germany, the outlook for patients with sino-venous thrombosis can be greatly improved by anticoagulant treatment especially if this can be given early, and that previous fears about the dangers of anticoagulants have been exaggerated. This further emphasizes the crucial relevance of early diagnosis and how important it is to be aware, not only of the many different ways in which venous disease may present, but also of the most relevant investigations and effective treatment.

1

Anatomy and Physiology of the Cerebral Venous System

The cerebral veins contain 70% of the total cerebral blood volume, and are arranged into a superficial and a deep venous system. The superficial veins on the surface of the brain drain the outer 2 cm of cerebral cortex and white matter, and lead into the major dural venous sinuses. The deep cerebral veins drain blood in a centripetal direction from deep hemisphere white matter, basal ganglia and diencephalon. They include subependymal veins, internal cerebral veins, basal veins, internal occipital veins and other smaller veins contributing to the great vein of Galen (Galenic system).

Within the cerebral substance, veins have a geometric disposition similar to arteries, running perpendicularly to the surface and each draining a hexagonal block of tissue via a system of horizontal post-capillary venules at various levels (Figure 1.1). There are numerous connections between adjacent veins on the pial surface but not within the cerebral substance (Figure 1.2). Occasional pre-capillary arterio-venous anastomoses are present (Duvernoy, 1977).

SUPERFICIAL VENOUS SYSTEM

Veins on the external convexity of the cerebral hemispheres are thin-walled with no defined muscle coat and no valves. There are three groups on each side: superior, middle and inferior. **Superior** veins number 8–12; they tend to run in the sulci and drain upwards towards the superior sagittal sinus (Figure 1.3). There are many individual variations and asymmetries, and the anatomy of the cerebral veins is much less uniform than that of the arteries.

Five cortical veins are usually larger than the rest and run in the prefrontal, precentral, central, post-central and parieto-occipital sulci. They anastomose with each other and with the middle cerebral veins. A prominent anastomosis in the central fissure (Trolard's vein) links the superior and middle venous systems (Figure 1.4). Veins draining the convexity of the frontal lobes show

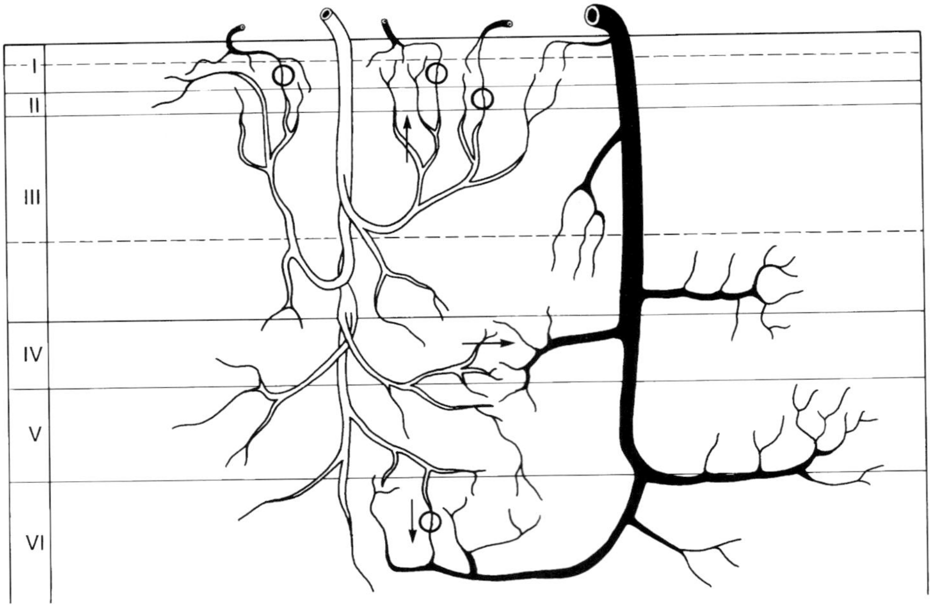

Figure 1.1 Typical arrangement of an intracortical artery and vein in human grey matter. Possible precapillary anastomoses are present in layers I and VI. The cortical cellular layers are shown on the left. Redrawn after Duvernoy (1977) with permission.

many variations. There are four main groups: fronto-polar, inferior frontal, middle frontal and superofrontal, and their arrangement depends on the state of development of the anterior portion of the superior sagittal sinus. If this is defective, a major vein may run in the superior frontal sulcus parallel to the sagittal sinus (Perese, 1960).

At the superio-medial border of each hemisphere the veins draining the convexity of the brain are joined by four equivalent tributaries draining the medial surface and the corpus callosum; anchor or bridge veins span the subarachnoid space and join the superior sagittal sinus.

The superficial **middle cerebral vein** originates near the posterior limb of the Sylvian fissure, and runs downwards and forward towards the pterion. It drains the Sylvian area and runs into the spheno-parietal sinus and finally into the cavernous sinus. There are usually four tributaries: middle superficial cerebral, temporal inferior, occipital inferior and anastomotic (Lang and Schneider, 1989). These show the greatest variability of all the cerebral veins and, if the sphenoido-parietal sinus is not well formed, they may drain directly into the transverse sinus via a series of small channels. The inferior anastomotic vein (Labbés vein) is an important venous collateral on the convexity of the hemisphere, which connects the middle cerebral vein to the transverse sinus (Figure 1.4).

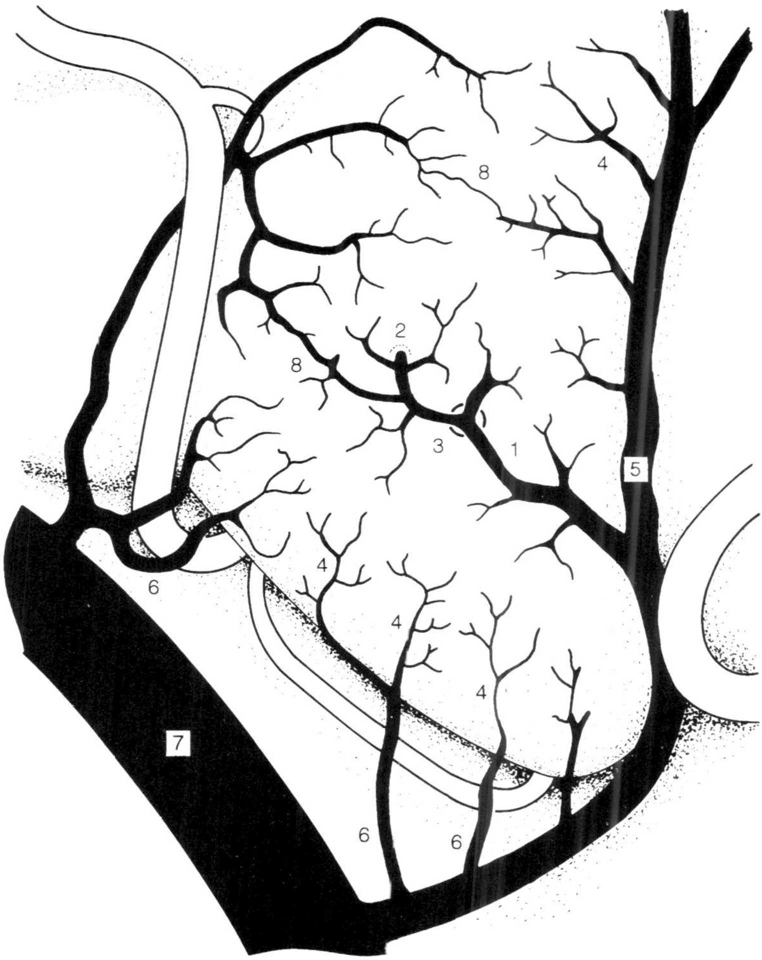

Figure 1.2 Pial veins on the surface of the cerebral cortex. The pial arteries have been removed. 1, Central vein of the gyrus; 2 and 3, junction point of intracortical and pial venules; 4, peripheral veins; 5, marginal vein; 6, the collecting veins of the pial network cross over the arteries and the sulcus to flow into the superficial cerebral vein; 7, superficial cerebral vein; 8, pial venous anastomoses. Redrawn after Duvernoy (1977) with permission.

The superficial **inferior cerebral veins** are smaller and drain the under surface of the hemispheres. Those in the frontal lobe drain into the superior sagittal sinus, those in the temporal lobe drain into the cavernous, petrosal and transverse sinuses.

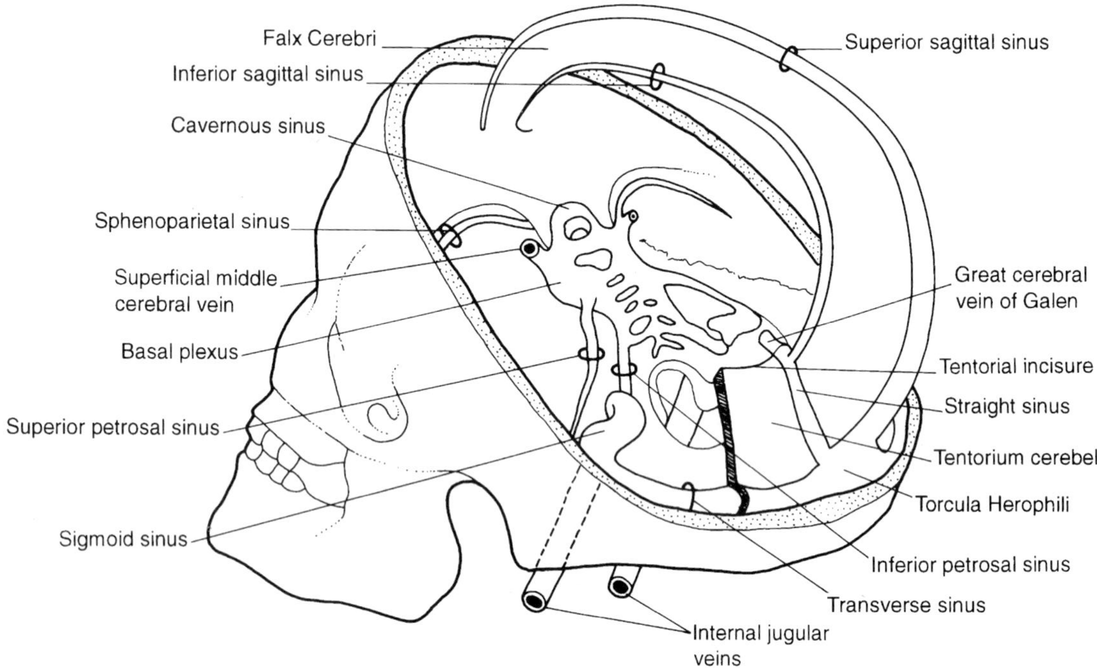

Figure 1.3 Base of skull and cerebral venous sinuses. Redrawn from Hausman, *Illustrations of the Central Nervous System* (1961). Courtesy of Charles C. Thomas, Publisher, Springfield, Illinois.

THE DEEP VENOUS SYSTEM

The **basal veins** (Rosenthal) are formed by the union of each anterior cerebral vein with the deep middle cerebral and striate veins. The basal vein runs round the cerebral peduncle and drains into the great cerebral vein, receiving tributaries from the inferior temporal lobe and mid-brain. The drainage area includes the temporal horn of the lateral ventricle including the dentate gyrus and hippocampus, inferior thalamus and hypothalamus, and the inter-peduncular fossa (Figures 1.4 and 1.5).

Two **internal cerebral veins** drain the deeper parts of the hemispheres. Each is formed by the union of the thalamo-striate vein draining the basal ganglia including the dorsal thalamus and the choroidal vein draining the choroid plexus, hippocampus, fornix and corpus callosum. In the region of the pineal gland, the two internal cerebral veins unite to form the **great cerebral vein** (of Galen) (Figure 1.6). The great cerebral vein is short and mid-line. It runs upwards in the region of the splenium, receives the two basal veins and joins the straight sinus.

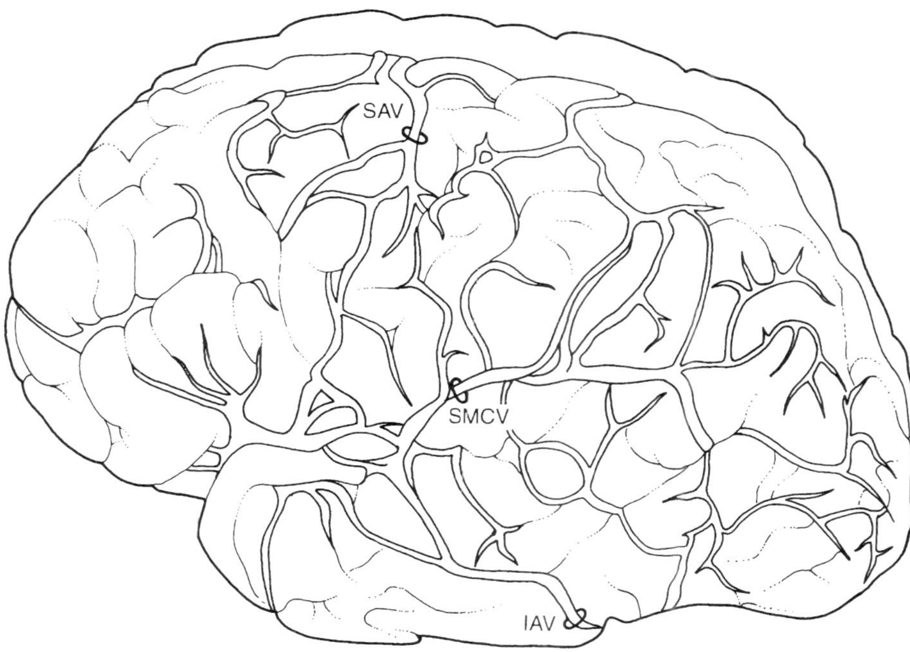

Figure 1.4 The superficial veins of the left cerebral hemisphere. The superior anastomotic vein (Trolard's vein) drains into the superior sagittal sinus, the superficial middle cerebral vein into the cavernous sinus and the inferior anastomotic vein (Labbe's vein) into the transverse sinus. Redrawn after Waddington (1974). SAV, superior anastomotic vein (Trolard). SMCV, superficial middle cerebral vein. IAV, inferior anastomotic vein (Labbé).

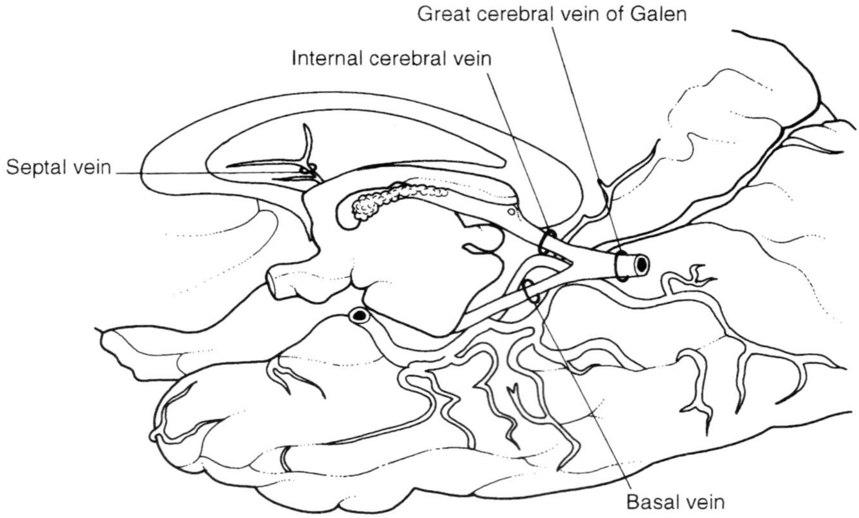

Figure 1.5 The left cerebral hemisphere, medial aspect, viewed from below showing the junction of the internal cerebral vein and the basal vein to form the great cerebral vein (of Galen). Redrawn after Waddington (1974).

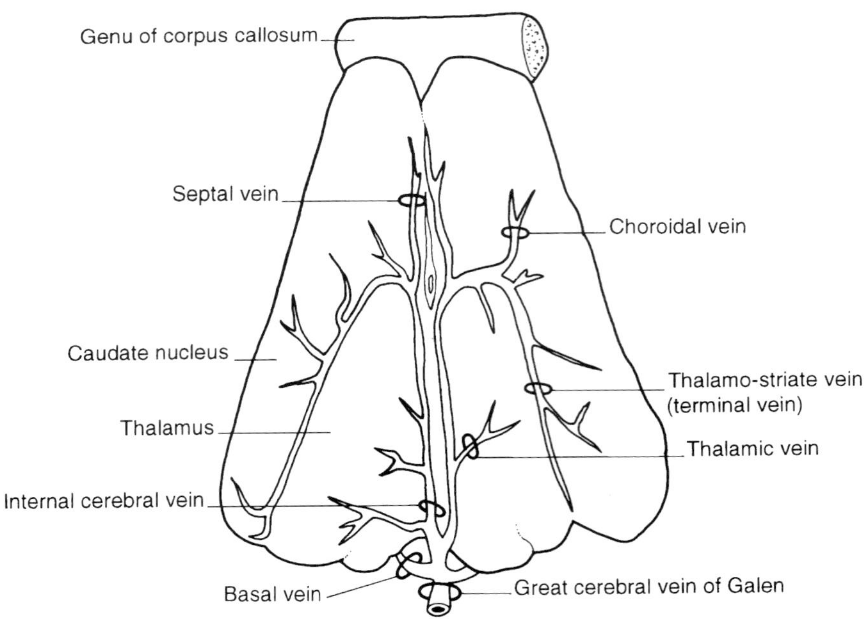

Figure 1.6 Thalami and caudate nuclei viewed from above (choroid plexus deleted) to show the deep cerebral veins. Redrawn after Waddington (1974).

VEINS OF THE CEREBELLUM AND BRAINSTEM

The superficial venous drainage of the cerebellum is regional into adjacent large veins and sinuses. The major outlets are the vein of Galen, the basal vein, the petrosal sinus, the straight sinus, the torcular and the transverse sinus. On the surface of the cerebellum the superficial veins form a coarse network and tend to run at right-angles to the folia. The cerebellar vermis and the adjacent superior surface drain into the superior vermian vein and precentral cerebellar vein, and finally into the vein of Galen (Figure 1.8). The petrosal and transverse

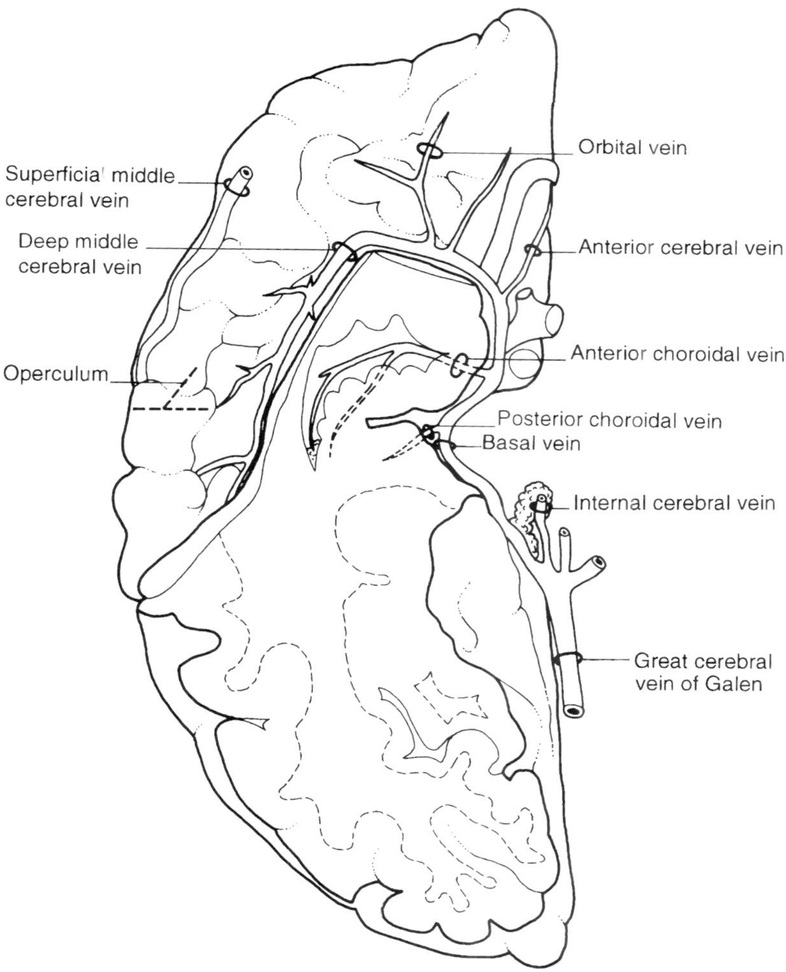

Figure 1.7 Inferior part of the deep cerebral veins, left cerebral hemisphere. Parts of the temporal lobe have been resected to show the deep middle cerebral vein and the anterior choroidal vein. Redrawn after Waddington (1974).

sinuses are the main route of venous blood from the laterally situated veins of both the superior and inferior cerebellar hemispheres (Figure 1.9). Many of the remaining veins from the surface of the cerebellum lead into the petrosal vein; they include tributaries from the precentral fissure, the cerebello-medullary fissure, the restiform body and the medial tonsillar vein.

The veins of the brainstem comprise a superior or Galenic group, an anterior or petrosal group, and a posterior or tentorial group. The superior group receives blood from the mid-brain via the tectal veins and the anterior, lateral and posterior ponto-mesencephalic veins. The petrosal group drains the anterior aspect of the mid-brain and pons via the anterior and lateral ponto-mesencephalic veins, the peduncular vein and the pontine veins.

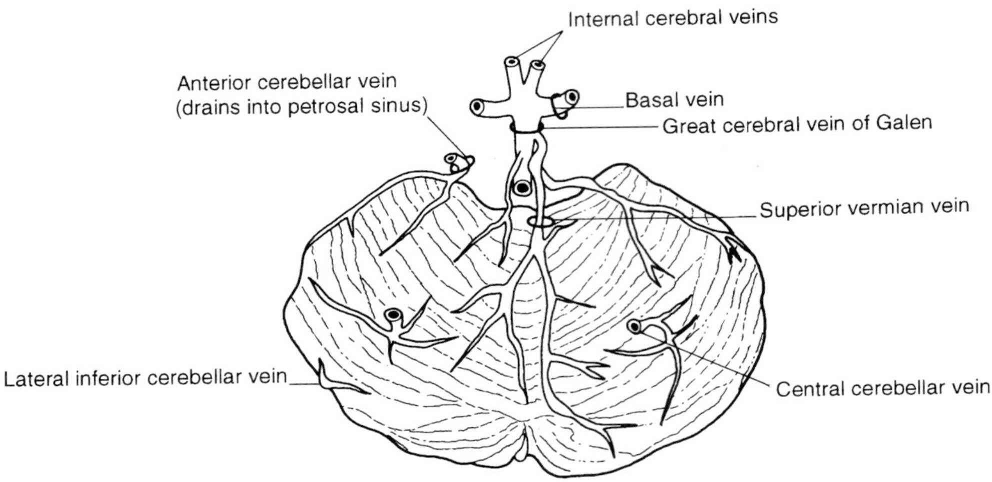

Figure 1.8 Veins of the posterior fossa. View of the superior surface of the cerebellum. Redrawn after Waddington (1974).

CEREBRAL VENOUS SINUSES

The venous sinuses are enclosed between fibrous layers of the dura mater, and are located at junctions and edges of the falx cerebri and the tentorium cerebelli. They receive tributaries from the superficial and deep venous systems as well as from the cranial vault via a system of venous lakes within the skull bones. Most of the cerebral venous blood flows posteriorly and drains via the sigmoid sinuses into internal jugular veins. A smaller proportion flows to the cavernous sinus, which has connections with the internal jugular vein and also with the pterygoid plexus. There are no valves in the venous sinuses.

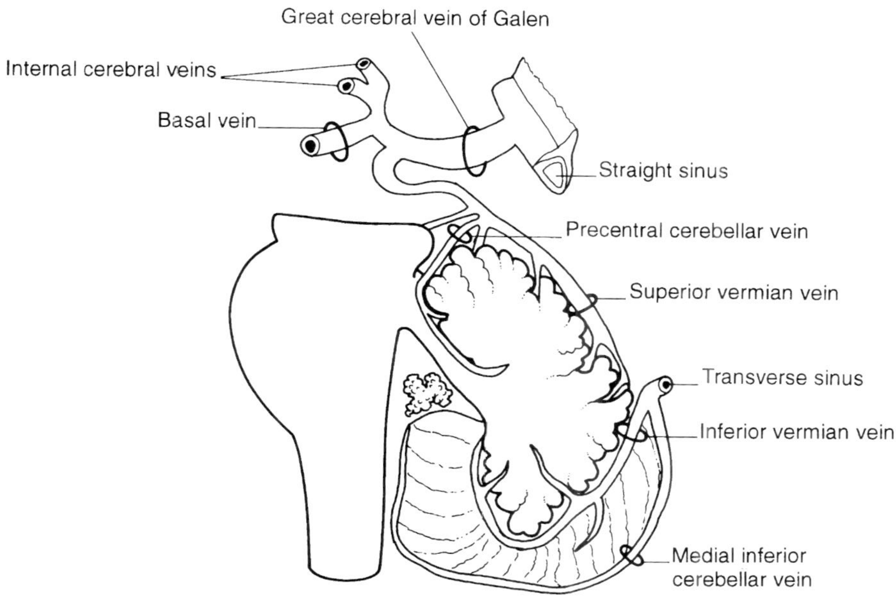

Figure 1.9 Mid-sagittal section of the cerebellum and brainstem to show the vermian and other cerebellar veins draining into the great vein of Galen and into the transverse sinus. Redrawn after Waddington (1974).

The **superior sagittal sinus** (Figure 1.3) begins near the foramen caecum and may connect with a caecal emissary vein. The sinus follows the falx cerebri towards the internal occipital protruberance. It is triangular in shape with the base attached to the inner table of the cranium. Lateral lacunae extend outwards on both sides of the sagittal sinus receiving blood from the diploic and meningeal veins. They are of very variable size and can be several centimetres long and up to 2.5 cm wide. There are three main lateral lacunae, frontal lacuna receiving the frontal cortical veins, the parietal receiving the pre- and post-central veins, and occipital receiving the occipital veins. Superficial cortical veins lie underneath the lacunae and either empty into them via openings in the floor or empty directly into the sagittal sinus.

At the internal occipital protuberance, the superior sagittal sinus takes a right-angled bend to terminate in most cases in the right transverse sinus. Considerable individual variation occurs in this area in the proportions of blood from the right and left side reaching the torcular (Woodhall, 1936). In a detailed study of 100 brains, there was a major disproportion between the size of the transverse sinuses in one quarter, with the right side usually being the larger and receiving blood from the superior sagittal sinus:

- In 13% the left side was the larger.
- In 4% one of the transverse sinuses was absent.

- In 5% the transverse sinus was replaced by an abnormal occipital sinus.
- In 10–15% there was inadequate cross-circulation at the torcular.
- In only 10% was there a common pool.
- In 56% there was a plexiform venous structure with persistence of the fetal vascular pattern.
- In 30% there was strictly ipsilateral drainage with a communicating foramen.

In the remainder there was either unilateral drainage with no right–left connection or a large occipital sinus, single or paired, which replaced the transverse sinuses. There are also variations in the origin of the sagittal sinus; instead of beginning at the foramen caecum there may be an atretic segment 2 mm–9 cm in extent. When this is present there are supplementary venous channels in the dura overlying the frontal lobes, which provide alternative pathways for venous drainage into the fully developed posterior portion of the sinus. Another not uncommon variant is duplication of the posterior third of the sinus.

The **inferior sagittal sinus** (Figure 1.3) runs in the free ventral edge of the falx cerebri, draining the corpus callosum, cingulate gyrus and medial part of the hemisphere. The **straight sinus** originates posterior to the splenium of the corpus callosum, and is formed by the union of the inferior sagittal sinus and vein of Galen, with contributions from the superior cerebellar veins and basal vein. It proceeds backwards and downwards in the junction of the falx and the tentorium cerebelli, and, at the internal occipital protuberance, it usually runs into the left transverse sinus or into the torcular. It may also communicate with the superior sagittal sinus. Doubling of portions of the straight sinus is a common variation, occurring in about 14% of brains.

Each **lateral sinus** (Figure 1.3) is made up of two portions, the transverse sinus and the sigmoid sinus. The **transverse sinus** starts at the torcular and passes laterally and anteriorly along the edges of the tentorium cerebelli in a groove in the squamous temporal bone. Much of the venous drainage of the cerebellum is into the transverse sinus: the superior cerebellum is drained via vessels running in the tentorium, inferior cerebellar veins join the sinus at a number of points and veins draining the anterior cerebellum empty into the distal part of the transverse sinus. An occipital emissary vein and the pterygo-squamous sinus may also join the transverse sinus at this point. As it leaves the tentorium cerebelli the transverse sinus receives the superior petrosal sinus and becomes the **sigmoid sinus**. This curves downwards and medially, grooving the mastoid portion of the temporal bone and in close relation to the mastoid air cells and tympanic antrum. Mastoid and condylar emissary veins connect the sigmoid sinus with pericranial veins. The sigmoid sinus is continuous with the superior bulb of the internal jugular vein and leaves the skull through the jugular foramen.

The **occipital sinus** is the smallest of the cerebral venous sinuses. It is formed by the union of the two marginal sinuses. It may be single, paired or occasionally absent and runs in the root of the falx cerebelli. It communicates with the internal vertebral venous plexus and ends in the torcular. If the transverse sinuses are poorly developed, the occipital sinus may constitute a major route of venous drainage from the brain. Large venous lakes communicating with the occipital sinus may be present in childhood. The torcular and major venous sinuses originate from a network of tentorial veins in the embryo.

There are numerous anatomical variations, particularly in the occipital region, and some of these are of clinical significance. The most important are:

1. Absence of the superior sagittal sinus and its replacement by paired frontal cortical veins (see above).
2. Duplication of the superior sagittal sinus or division by a mid-line septum. This is commonest in its posterior segment and separation may be partial or complete.
3. Asymmetry of the transverse sinuses (see above). Communication between right and left sides at the torcula is highly variable, and in some cases there may be no mixing of blood from superficial and deep venous systems.
4. The straight sinus may join the torcular, the right transverse sinus, the left transverse sinus or both. Most often it opens to the left side.
5. There is complete or incomplete septation of the transverse sinus with hypoplasia of its proximal part. Another variant is irregular narrowing of the transverse sinus by a cavernous nodule or dural venous pouch at the point of junction with the anastomotic vein of Labbé. This may result in draining of Labbés vein to the contralateral side.
6. Labbés vein may drain into the superior sagittal sinus rather than into the transverse sinus.

There are a number of venous sinuses draining the anterior parts of the brain. Of these, the most important are the **cavernous sinuses** (Figure 1.13) on each side of the basisphenoid and in close relation to the pituitary gland and carotid arteries. These sinuses are spongy structures interlaced by fine septa and often communicating with one another across the mid-line. Tributaries of the cavernous sinus are the ophthalmic veins, spheno-parietal sinuses, superficial middle cerebral veins and a variable number of inferior cerebral veins (Figure 1.3). There are also communications between the cavernous sinus, the anterior facial vein and the pterygoid and basilar plexuses. From the cavernous sinus blood passes either via the superior petrosal sinus to the transverse sinus or directly via the inferior petrosal sinus to the internal jugular vein. **Petrosal sinuses**, (Figure 1.3) superior and inferior, both communicate anteriorly with the cavernous sinus. The superior runs in the margin of the tentorium cerebelli, the inferior in relation to the petro-occipital suture. The superior sinus drains the under surface of the temporal lobes and the superior surface of the cerebellum. It also receives the petrosal vein and the lateral mesencephalic vein. It is closely related to the Gasserian ganglion. It terminates in the proximal part of the

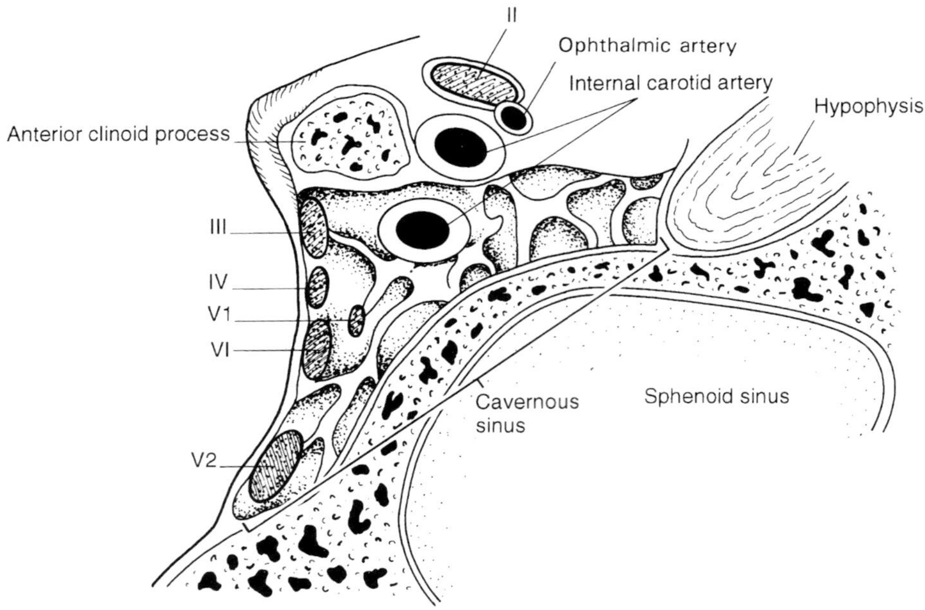

Figure 1.10 Coronal section through right cavernous sinus, detailing structures within sinus cavity itself. II, indicates optic nerve; III, oculomotor nerve; IV, trochlear nerve; V, trigeminal nerve: V1, ophthalmic branch; V2, maxillary branch; and VI, abducens nerve. Redrawn from DiNubile, Septic thrombosis of the cavernous sinuses. Neurological review. *Archives of Neurology* **38:** 431–435 (1988). Courtesy of the AMA, Chicago, Illinois.

sigmoid sinus. The inferior petrosal sinus passes underneath the petroclinoid ligament and receives branches from the undersurface of the cerebellum, the brainstem and the internal auditory veins. There are connections between the two inferior petrosal sinuses via the basilar plexus, a network of venous channels lying between the two layers of dura over the basi-occiput and also indirect connections with the marginal sinus and vertebral venous plexus (Figure 1.3). The inferior petrosal sinuses drain directly or indirectly into the internal jugular vein, or sometimes into the deep cervical veins.

Emissary veins are bridging veins between the dural sinuses and veins outside the skull. They are of clinical importance as potential routes of infection and spread of thrombosis after injury. They include: (1) the mastoid emissary running in the mastoid foramen, and connecting the sigmoid sinus and the occipital vein; (2) the anterior condylar emissary vein connecting the marginal sinus, jugular bulb and vertebral venous plexus; (3) the posterior condylar emissary connecting the jugular bulb to the occipital vein or to the external vertebral venous plexus; (4) the occipital emissary vein connecting the torcular to the occipital and posterior jugular veins; and (5) a number of parietal emissaries, which empty into the superior sagittal sinus. The existence of a rostral caecal emissary into the sagittal sinus has been questioned.

PHYSIOLOGY OF THE CEREBRAL VENOUS SYSTEM

The structure of the venous sinuses, lying enclosed by folds of fibrous dura, ensures that they do not collapse but remain open at all times, even when transmural pressure is zero. Cerebral veins do not have this rigid structure but they too remain open in the face of zero intravascular pressure. This is because a transmural pressure gradient is maintained by a negative intracranial pressure within the closed cranial cavity. The cerebral veins are also protected from collapse when intracranial pressure rises. Within physiological limits a rise in intracranial pressure causes dilatation of arteries as part of the autoregulatory response. Venous calibre remains unaltered because a parallel rise in intracranial and venous pressure keeps the venous transmural pressure constant.

Changes in blood pressure cause the vessels to react in a similar manner. Systemic hypotension is followed by a marked autoregulatory dilatation in large arteries on the brain surface but there is little change in the veins. Hypertension results in arterial constriction alone. Auer *et al.* (1987) using video angiometry on the pial veins of the cat found that venous calibre remained unaltered within a range of 40–160 mm systemic pressure.

The unusual physical properties of the cerebral venous system have been examined in the Starling resistor model (Holt, 1941) in which flow through collapsible tubes is studied within a rigid fluid-filled container. The Starling theorem states that, as long as flow is maintained, intravascular pressure and perivascular pressures are almost equal. This explains why veins remain open over a wide range of transmural pressures and why venous capacitance remains relatively constant. In real life small changes in capacitance can in fact be achieved by changing the cross-sectional area of the large veins from elliptical to circular or by contraction of the small numbers of smooth muscle cells present in venous walls.

Neurigenic responses similar or greater in degree to those seen in cerebral arteries have been measured in pial veins following sympathetic nerve stimulation and histochemical or immunofluorescent techniques have shown adrenergic nerve fibres, derived from the cervical sympathetic trunk, in the walls of large and small cerebral veins. Adrenergic responses are abolished by alpha blockade. Pial veins also react to topically applied vaso-active substances. Noradrenaline causes constriction, and vasoactive peptide or substance P cause dilatation in both arteries and veins. Although large collecting veins also have perivascular nerve fibres, they may react differently to smaller veins. Serotonin or papaverine appear to dilate small arteries and veins, but constrict larger arteries and have no effect on large veins. Similarly hypocapnia constricts small veins and arteries, but produces no change in larger vessels.

The relative insensitivity of cerebral veins as compared to arteries to changes in pH and potassium concentration was shown by McCulloch *et al.* (1982). A rise in potassium concentration in the perivascular fluid, for instance, caused a dilatation of 47% in arteries but only 14% in veins. The authors suggest that humoral changes in the perivascular space are of lesser importance in the control of capacitance than of resistance vessels.

As the veins merge into larger collecting channels on the surface of the brain, laminar flow from each tributary is often preserved. In the pial intervenous anastomoses, flow is irregular and slow, sometimes stagnant, reversing or oscillating. Changes in the direction of venous flow are a particular feature of the cerebral circulation, on account of the absence of venous valves.

2

Pathology and Pathogenesis of Venous Infarction

CONSEQUENCES OF VENOUS OCCLUSION

Not every vein occlusion is followed by infarction; this will only occur if venous pressure rises sufficiently to lower cerebral perfusion pressure (arterio-venous difference) below the limit of autoregulation and so reduce cerebral blood flow below the critical level necessary for neuronal survival.

There are two main factors that determine the outcome of venous occlusion: the availability of pre-existing collateral venous channels and the extent to which the thrombus propagates along the veins. Other compensatory mechanisms such as formation of new venous collaterals (neo-vascularization) occur too slowly to have an influence on early infarction.

On the brain surface there are pial collaterals that link adjacent veins and, in addition, there are larger channels (the anastomotic veins of Trolard and Labbé) connecting superior, middle and inferior venous systems. Experimental and neurosurgical observations indicate that these provide adequate alternative routes for venous drainage following blockage of any of the large pial veins provided that only a short segment of vein is occluded. However, should thrombosis spread along the vein to occlude anastomotic channels, the possibility of cerebral damage is much increased. Similarly, in the case of venous sinus thrombosis, the effects in terms of infarction depend on the site and the extent of occlusion, and on the adequacy of venous collateral channels.

Gotoh *et al.* (1993) studied the effects of experimental sinus and cortical vein occlusion in the cat, measuring intracranial pressure, cerebral blood volume and regional cerebral blood flow for periods up to 12 hours. Occlusion of the sagittal sinus produced an immediate rise in intracranial pressure and blood volume, and a decrease in regional cerebral blood flow. There was an increase in brain water content but no visible leakage of vital dyes from the veins. Leakage, indicating a severe breakdown of the blood–brain barrier, only occurred when the superficial cortical veins or bridging veins were also occluded. These results have been confirmed in other species using a variety of methods to occlude the veins (Fries *et al.*, 1992).

Measurements of intracranial and venous pressure, and the occurrence of infarction following occlusion of the major venous channels in man have given broadly similar results. Lam *et al.* (1992) documented a rise in pressure in the sagittal sinus in five patients, two after unilateral dissection of cervical lymph nodes, one after surgical ligation of the dominant sigmoid sinus and two after catheterization of the internal jugular vein. Less than half of the cases of sagittal sinus thrombosis reported by Noetzel and Jerusalem (1965) showed cerebral infarction; six out of 17 patients reported by Merwarth (1942) showed no clinical sequelae following ligation of the sagittal sinus in its anterior third and, of 23 cases of sinus thrombosis without extension to cortical veins studied by Cervos-Navarro and Kannuki (1990), 20 showed no pathological changes in the brain. Ligation of the sinus posterior to the entry of the Rolandic veins, however, was more likely to be followed by infarction. The rate of occlusion is a further important factor; in cases where the sinus is slowly narrowed by growth of adjacent tumour there is more time for the development of collaterals and less likelihood of parenchymal damage. By contrast, rapid thrombosis, or ligation of superficial cortical veins or deep cerebral veins is much more likely to be followed by infarction, often haemorrhagic in type.

Pre-existing collateral venous channels often show a progressive enlargement following vein occlusion, apparently in response to an increased blood flow. In some cases, this may go on to the formation of an arterio-venous fistula and a dural arterio-venous malformation (see below). There is some doubt as to the origin of the spiral collateral channels, which may appear within the cerebral parenchyma after extensive thrombosis of the superficial veins. Some regard them as enlarged pre-existing venous channels and some as new vessels derived from the capillary bed. Kaplan (1959), in support of the first suggestion, has described in the normal brain a system of small veins running parallel to the fibres of the corona radiata, which he terms the transcerebral venous system. When dilated and acting as collaterals, these veins have a characteristic morphology and can be recognized on angiography as delicate spiral structures running in cerebral white matter and usually draining into the deep cerebral venous system.

PATHOLOGY OF VENOUS INFARCTION

Cerebral venous infarction is the result of ischaemia and is characterized macroscopically by pallor, and oedema of cortex and white matter in the territory drained by a thrombosed vein (Figures 2.1, 2.2 and 2.3). In addition there are multiple petechial haemorrhages, which may become confluent, especially in white matter. Special features that distinguish venous from arterial infarction are distended and thrombosed sinuses and cortical veins,

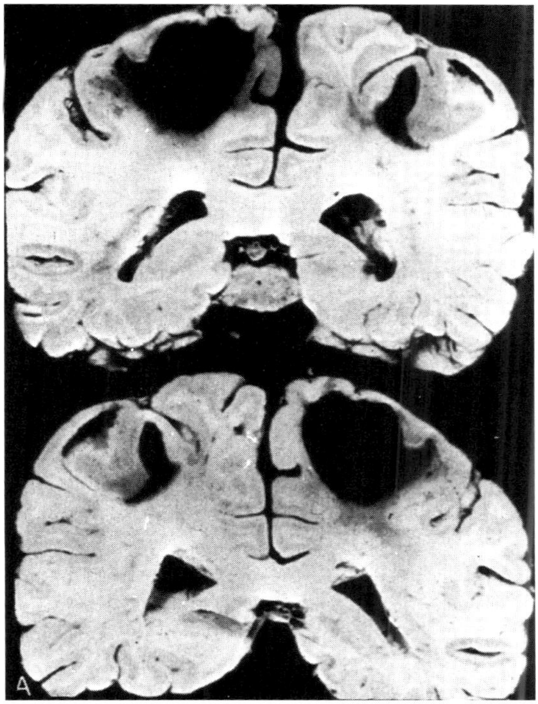

Figure 2.1 Typical appearance of haemorrhagic bilateral venous infarcts in the posterior parietal region secondary to thrombosis of the superior sagittal sinus. (By courtesy of Professor F. Scaravilli, National Hospital, London.)

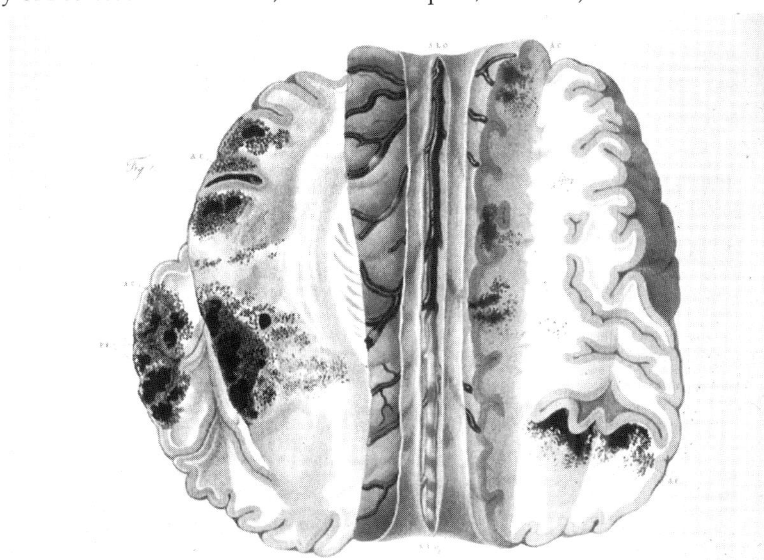

Figure 2.2 An illustration from Cruveilhier's Atlas (1829) showing thrombus of various ages in the superior sagittal sinus with bilateral haemorrhagic infarction of the cerebral cortex.

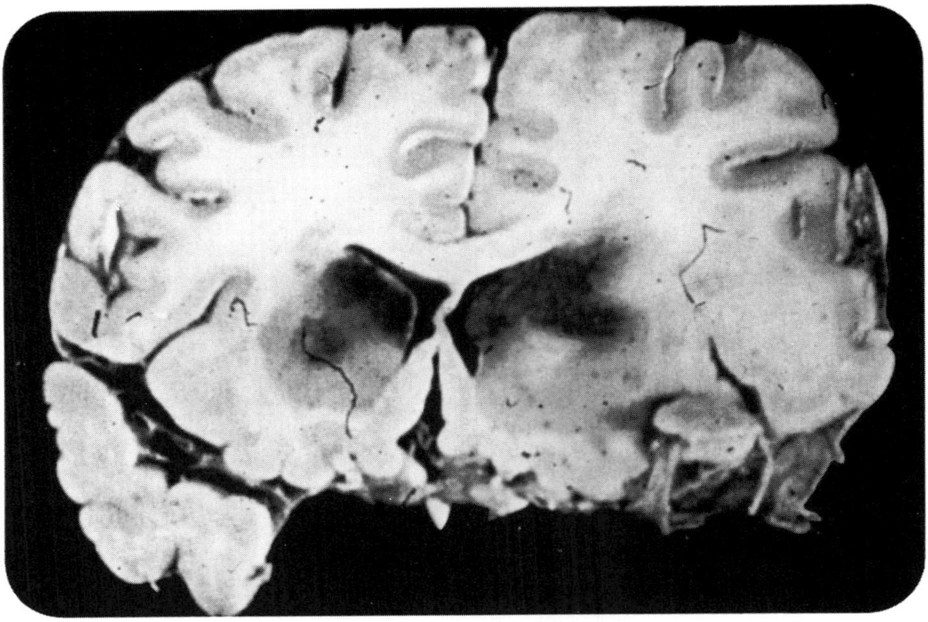

Figure 2.3 Bilateral haemorrhagic infarction of the basal ganglia as a result of thrombosis of the deep venous system. (Reproduced with permission from Waddington (1974), Little Brown, Boston.)

often with perivenous subarachnoid haemorrhage on the brain surface, and sometimes with larger areas of subdural haemorrhage. The gyri are flattened from cerebral swelling (Cobb and Hubbard, 1929; Bucy and Lesemann, 1942). Because of the wide variation in the territories of cortical veins, the extent and location of venous infarcts are less uniform than those resulting from arterial occlusion.

Histological changes reflect mainly ischaemic damage; there are early changes in neurones with loss of staining of the cytoplasm and pyknotic nuclei and, at a later stage, the number of neurones is greatly reduced. Oligodendrocytes show vacuolar cytoplasmic swelling, there is intense congestion of venules with numerous haemorrhages, and swelling and hypertrophy of endothelial cells. There may be profuse neutrophil infiltration of the cerebral parenchyma. The surrounding regions, which have escaped severe ischaemia, show some loss of neurones with astrocytic and microglial proliferation, and spongy change in the neurophil. Club-like processes, thought to be derived from interrupted axis cylinders, are a prominent feature of venous infarction in infancy and childhood, and recanalized veins are numerous. At a later stage necrotic cortex and white matter disintegrate leaving a shrunken cystic brownish scar.

INTRAVASCULAR THROMBOSIS

Thrombosis within a cerebral vein or sinus is a dynamic process in which the tendency to thrombosis is held in check by the natural anticoagulant and thrombolytic properties of the blood. If thrombosis predominates, there is a tendency for the thrombus to propagate forwards or backwards from the point of origin (Garcin and Pestel, 1949), and in some cases thrombosis may occur simultaneously at a number of different sites. If lysis of the thrombus does not take place immediately, older parts of the thrombus may become organized and attached to the venous wall, while fresh thrombus may remain free within the lumen.

The various stages in the histological evolution of a thrombus within a cerebral vein or sinus have been more recently studied in a series of 41 fatal cases by Cervos-Navarro and Kannuki (1990). In brains examined within 2–3 days of clinical onset, recent platelet thrombi were found adherent to the venous endothelium. The platelets rapidly became aggregated and degranulated, and infiltrated with polymorphonuclear leucocytes. A laminated structure was evident from an early stage with layers of platelets alternating with layers of fibrin and entrapped red cells. Thrombus examined at 5–10 days showed a more homogeneous and hyalinized appearance with loss of cellular outlines and loss of the fibrillary structure of fibrin. At a still later stage (8–20 days), there were signs of organization of thrombus, and invasion by fibroblasts and capillaries. Spaces appeared in the thrombus by a process of retraction or lysis, and these became lined with endothelium. Endothelium also covered any surface of the thrombus exposed to the bloodstream. Gradually the whole thrombus became replaced by vascularized connective tissue and converted into a dense fibrous mass. In some places there was retraction of the thrombus from the original wall of the vein with reconstitution of a lumen. In cases examined at a late stage there was often evidence of thrombosis at various stages of evolution. There is evidence that in some cases there is rapid and complete lysis of thrombus without organization, and resulting in a normal-looking vein or sinus. Organization of thrombus is said to take place slowly in adults but rapidly in children. In general, the process occurs later in veins of the brain than in other organs.

Similar findings were published by Poltera (1972) on two patients dying of cerebral venous infarction following the use of oral contraceptive drugs. There was widespread thrombosis of the sagittal sinus and cortical veins. Laminated fresh thrombus was found adherent to the vessel walls, which showed oedema but no inflammation. Oedema and endothelial proliferation were prominent in the lateral lacunae and it was suggested that thrombosis started there, spreading later to sinus and cortical veins.

Pulmonary embolism as a potentially fatal complication of cerebral sinus thrombosis was well known to pathologists in the last century but has received little recent attention. In a large review of 203 cases from 1942 to 1990, Diaz *et al.*

(1992) found 11% to be associated with pulmonary embolism and, in these, the mortality rate was 49%. Anticoagulation appeared to lessen the risk of embolism.

In thrombosis secondary to infection, the thrombus is infiltrated with inflammatory cells, which may also be present in large numbers in the walls of the veins or sinuses. An organizing infective thrombus may show multiple microabscesses (Doyle, 1927).

The site of thrombosis within the cerebral venous system was studied by Huhn (1965) (see also Table 3.3). As expected, in cases secondary to infection, Huhn found that the affected vein or sinus was the vessel draining the infected region. In aseptic thrombosis, however, the superior sagittal sinus appeared to be the most susceptible. In 36 observations, there were 24 examples of thrombosis at this site and in 19 of these the lateral sinus was also involved (14 had bilateral lateral sinus thrombosis). In four cases only the lateral sinus was affected. Thrombosis of the inferior sagittal sinus, the petrosal sinus and the straight sinus was exceptional. There were 34 examples of thrombosis of surface veins, but in only seven of these were the sinuses free of thrombus. Sixteen showed asymmetrical involvement of both sides and in only three was the thrombosis entirely unilateral. The Galenic system was involved in seven cases, all occurring in infants and all associated with widespread thrombosis in other sites.

EFFECTS ON CEREBROSPINAL FLUID CIRCULATION

Aside from venous infarction, the main effects of venous thrombosis are interference with cerebrospinal fluid (CSF) circulation and cranial nerve palsies. Intracranial hypertension is caused by impaired CSF absorption either from blockage of arachnoid granulations by thrombus or from chronic raised venous pressure. The occurrence of intracranial hypertension usually indicates thrombosis of the superior sagittal sinus. Lateral sinus thrombosis, a complication of sepsis in the middle ear or mastoid region, tends to give rise to intracranial hypertension only if the thrombus extends back to involve the torcular or if there is poor communication between left and right sides at the torcular.

The flow of cerebrospinal fluid into the superior sagittal sinus takes place at the arachnoid granulations where finger-like processes of arachnoid (arachnoid villi) project through the walls of the venous sinus and lateral lacunae. Endothelial cells covering the villi have prominent vesicular holes directly through the cell bodies, large enough to allow relatively free bulk flow of cerebrospinal fluid, including protein molecules and perhaps red cells, into venous blood. The rate of formation of CSF is constant and the villi function like valves, allowing flow in one direction only. The valves open at a pressure difference of 1.5 mm water and the degree of opening is proportional to the pressure difference. Blockage of the endothelial holes by particles, fibrosis or thrombosis, or by protein molecules leads to an increase in CSF pressure. Both experimental and clinical observations indicate that any type of obstruction of the sagittal sinus is sufficient to lead to increased CSF pressure. It is not necessary for the sinus to undergo thrombosis (Caudill *et al.*, 1953). Bedford (1935) carried out some of the first experimental studies on the effect of increased venous pressure on CSF pressure. He showed that occlusion of jugular vein or lateral sinus in the cat led to an immediate increase in CSF pressure, which then slowly declined over hours as the capacity of the collateral circulation increased. He also showed that the sinus pressure and the CSF pressure did not always correspond, and that high pressure in the torcular was compatible with a normal CSF pressure.

Mural thrombosis resulting in a thick mat of fibrin over the endothelium of the sagittal sinus was put forward by Symonds (1944) as an explanation of those cases in which intracranial hypertension occurred without complete obstruction of the sinus. It also appears that a rise in sinus pressure without actual thrombosis may be sufficient to impede CSF absorption. This is the mechanism suggested in some patients with arterio-venous fistulas adjacent to the sagittal sinus who may develop raised intracranial pressure without evidence of venous occlusion (Cockerwell *et al.*, 1993).

3

Clinical Features

SYMPTOMS AND SIGNS

The classical early accounts of cerebral venous thrombosis (CVT) were based on findings at autopsy. Bilateral or alternating focal deficits, seizures and coma were then described as constant features. In the last 30 years, the verification of the diagnosis during life has become possible and, as a result, the clinical spectrum of the disease has greatly increased. It is now well established that the clinical features of CVT are extraordinarily variable and that this variability depends on many factors such as the site and extent of thrombosis, the rate at which venous occlusion occurs, the age of the patient and the nature of any underlying disease, particularly the presence or absence of infection. The site and extent of thrombosis are important in determining whether or not infarction will occur and, in the case of superior sagittal sinus (SSS) or lateral sinus (LS), whether raised intracranial pressure will develop. When thrombosis affects a cerebral vein, an infarct will frequently develop with subsequent focal signs: these may be 'negative', such as a localized hemiparesis, or 'positive', such as a Jacksonian seizure. By contrast, when thrombosis is restricted to SSS or LS, focal signs are absent and the usual pattern is that of intracranial hypertension. The rate of thrombosis is an important factor in the evolution of venous infarction. It may be abrupt and stroke-like or it may be gradual, allowing time for the development of alternative pathways for venous drainage, which may protect against venous infarction or limit its extent. The presence of infection is often more life-threatening than the thrombosis itself and carries the possibility of widespread dissemination by septic embolism.

CVT presents with a remarkably wide spectrum of symptoms and signs as illustrated in Tables 3.1 and 3.2. Some are relatively specific for the location of thrombosis, such as painful ophthalmoplegia for cavernous sinus thrombosis, but many, such as headache or coma, are not specific and can occur whatever the location of thrombosis.

Table 3.1 Main neurologic signs and symptoms in 110 patients with cerebral venous thrombosis (from Ameri and Bousser, 1992)

Headache	83 (75%)
Papilloedema	54 (49%)
Motor or sensory deficit	38 (34%)
Seizures	41 (37%)
Drowsiness, mental changes, confusion or coma	33 (30%)
Dysphasia	13 (12%)
Multiple cranial nerve palsies	13 (12%)
Cerebellar incoordination	3 (3%)
Nystagmus	2 (2%)
Hearing loss	2 (2%)
Bilateral or alternating cortical signs	3 (3%)

HEADACHE

Headache is in all series the most frequent symptom of CVT. It is far more frequent than in patients with arterial cerebrovascular disease. It is probably caused by two main factors: the increased intracranial pressure, and the local involvement of the pain-sensitive fibres of the dura mater by distension of the sinus wall, local inflammation or leakage of blood on the surface of the brain.

Headache is the most frequent symptom, present in about 80% of reported cases (Tables 3.1 and 3.2). This is likely to be an underestimate because some comatose or aphasic patients might not have been able to report their headache. Headache is also the most frequent presenting symptom: 70% in Ameri and Bousser's series of 110 cases (1992, 1993), 73% in 67 puerperial cases and 61% in 46 non-puerperial cases in the series of Cantu and Barinagarrementeria (1993). Headache has no specific features: it can be of any grade of severity, it is slightly more frequently diffuse (58%) than localized (42%) (Ameri and Bousser, 1992, 1993). It is mostly persistent but can occasionally be intermittent. It is typically worse on recumbency and present on waking. It is aggravated by a short-term rise in venous pressure as in stooping or coughing. Its onset is usually subacute over a few days but it can also be acute (< 48 h) or chronic (> 30 days), respectively in 16% and 13% in Ameri's series (1993). It may be abrupt enough to suggest rupture of a berry aneurysm (Bousser *et al.*, 1985). It can even be mistaken for migraine because of unilaterality, intermittent course and associated visual phenomena mimicking an aura (Newman *et al.*, 1989). The most striking feature about headache in CVT is its association with other neurological signs. These were present in 94% of Ameri's series (1992–1993): focal signs (deficits or seizures) in 56% and papilloedema in 38%. However, in five patients, no other sign was present and CVT was discovered at systematic investigations for an isolated recent persisting headache.

Table 3.2 Main clinical signs in a recent series of patients with CVT

Signs	Einhaupl *et al.* (1990) ($n = 71$)	Ameri and Bousser (1992) ($n = 110$)	Cantu and Barrinagarrementeria (1993)		Tsai *et al.* (1995) ($n = 29$)	Daif *et al.* (1995) ($n = 40$)
			Puerperal ($n = 67$)	Non-puerperal ($n = 46$)		
Headache	91%	75%	88%	70%	31%	82%
Papilloedema	27%	49%	40%	52%	7%	80%
Focal deficits	66%	34%	79%	76%	31%	27%
Seizures	48%	37%	60%	63%	10%	10%
Altered consciousness	56%	30%	63%	59%	93%	10%

PAPILLOEDEMA

Papilloedema is present in about 50% of patients with CVT, the extremes being 15% (Krayenbühl, 1967) and 70% (Daif *et al.*, 1995) (Table 3.2). It tends to occur in young subjects: 56% in subjects below 45 years of age, 33% in Ameri and Bousser's series of 110 patients (1992, 1993). It is more frequent in subacute and chronic cases (56 and 35%, respectively) than in acute cases (6%), and in puerperal rather than in non-puerperal CVT (Cantu and Barinagarrementeria 1993). It has long been recognized as a constant finding in CVT due to Behçet's disease (Bousser *et al.*, 1980; Pamir *et al.*, 1981).

Papilloedema can be associated with bilateral transient amaurosis (visual obscurations) lasting a few seconds, and occurring at times of raised venous pressure or reduced arterial pressure as when stooping down or rapidly rising from the lying to the standing position. This symptom is usually found with high-grade papilloedema with microinfarcts on the discs and surrounding small-vessel engorgement or haemorrhages. In the early stages, visual acuity is unaffected and the visual fields are normal apart from enlargement of the blind spots, but if raised intracranial pressure persists untreated for weeks or months, the discs may become pale and there may be generalized field constriction especially in the infero-nasal quadrants. Central visual acuity is maintained until a late stage but finally field constriction encroaches on central vision. If untreated, the patient may eventually become completely blind (Bousser *et al.*, 1985; Ameri and Bousser, 1992; Daif *et al.*, 1995).

SEIZURES

Seizures are much more frequent than in arterial cerebro-vascular disease. They are inaugural in 12–15% of cases in Cantu's series (1993) and are present at some time during the course of CVT in about 40% of cases (from 10% to 61%) (Table 3.2). They signify an irritative cortical lesion and can occur in any region, although they are more frequent when the lesion is anterior to the central sulcus. Seizures are about equally divided between focal and generalized, and the association of both types is very common. They are rare and purely generalized when patients present with isolated intracranial hypertension. By contrast, they are frequent in patients who have focal deficits and, in some cases, seizures are followed by the appearance or aggravation of such focal signs. Repeated seizures and focal status epilepticus may occur, and may be difficult to control.

DISORDERS OF CONSCIOUSNESS

Alteration of consciousness is rarely an initial symptom [4% in Cantu's series (1993)] but is present during the course of the disease in about half the patients (Table 3.2). It is usually moderate in degree, varying from slight loss of alertness to somnolence and irritability. It is frequently associated with headache and papilloedema and is mainly caused by raised intracranial pressure. Deep unconsciousness is unusual except as a post-ictal event or as a sign of deep venous system thrombosis with bilateral thalamic involvement. Although the decreased level of consciousness found in CVT is usually reversible, it indicates a poor prognosis (Barinagarrementeria *et al.*, 1992). In Ameri's series (1992), death or sequelae were observed in 38% of cases with disorders of consciousness and in 16% of those with normal consciousness ($p < 0.02$).

FOCAL DEFICITS

Focal deficits are inaugural in about 15% of cases (Cantu *et al.*, 1993) and are present at some time during the course of the disease in about 60% of the cases (Table 3.2). The type of deficit varies with the site and extent of thrombosis: the most frequent are motor and sensory deficits, usually unilateral and often predominating in the leg. Occasionally, CVT can present as paraplegia mimicking a spinal disorder. Other symptoms include aphasia, cranial nerve palsies, and cerebellar signs. Among cranial nerve palsies, some are suggestive of a particular site of thrombosis, such as total ophthalmoplegia for cavernous sinus thrombosis, ninth and tenth nerve palsies for internal jugular vein thrombosis. By contrast, a unilateral or bilateral abducens nerve palsy is common in raised intracranial pressure and has then no localizing value. It is thought to be caused by traction on the sixth nerve in its long course through the subarachnoid space.

MODES OF ONSET

By contrast to arterial stroke, which almost always occurs abruptly, CVT has a variable mode of onset. In most series, a gradual development of symptoms is more common than a sudden onset. Three modes of onset have been arbitrarily defined: acute (symptoms appear suddenly or develop in less than 48 hours), subacute (more than 48 hours but less than 30 days), and chronic (progression during more than 30 days). An acute onset was found in 28% of cases in Ameri's (1992) series of 110 patients, in 35% of Daif's series of 40 patients (1995), and in 54% in Cantu's series (1993) of 46 non-puerperal cases and in 82% of 67 puerperal cases. An acute onset is thus frequent in obstetric CVT. This is also the case in infectious CVT, whereas a chronic or subacute onset is more frequent in inflammatory diseases and in idiopathic cases (Ameri and Bousser, 1992). Acute cases are often characterized by the presence of focal signs whereas in chronic cases headache is often the leading symptom. A subacute onset was observed in 42% of cases in Ameri's series (1992) and in 40% in Daif's series (1995). A chronic onset was respectively observed in 30% and 25%. Occasionally symptoms can progress insidiously over more than 6 months [8% in Bousser *et al.*'s series (1985)].

PATTERNS OF PRESENTATION

With such a wide spectrum of neurologic signs and such a variable mode of onset, CVT can present in a number of different ways and can mimic numerous other conditions.

ISOLATED INTRACRANIAL HYPERTENSION

Isolated intracranial hypertension is the most homogeneous pattern, accounting for up to 40% of cases of CVT (Ameri and Bousser, 1992). It is mainly characterized by headache and papilloedema, which are almost invariably present, usually in combination. There are, however, some rare cases of headache without papilloedema leading to great diagnostic difficulties. The clue is to perform neuroimaging investigations whenever headache is recent and progressing. Occasionally the reverse situation is encountered: papilloedema is present in the absence of headache. The diagnostic difficulty then is to rule out the other causes of bilateral papilloedema without visual loss, such as optic nerve drusen. The measurement of CSF pressure is necessary when there is doubt between drusen and papilloedema.

Other signs are less frequent and include horizontal diplopia from VIth nerve palsy, transient visual obscurations, nausea and vomiting, mild cognitive impairment with decreased concentration and loss of alertness, especially during headache. Consciousness is occasionally depressed. Such a presentation resembles that of benign intracranial hypertension (BIH) (pseudotumour cerebri), first described by Symonds (1940) under the term 'otitic hydrocephalus'. It occurs mainly in SSS and LS thrombosis. As in BIH, computed tomography (CT) brain scan shows either no abnormality or slight generalized brain swelling with reduced ventricular size. Distension of the optic nerve sheaths may be visible on axial and coronal views. Occasionally an empty delta sign is present, allowing a diagnosis of SSS thrombosis. Measurement of intracranial pressure by lumbar puncture confirms elevated pressure of 200–600 mm water; the constituents are normal unless there has been infarction or meningeal infiltration. The clinical, CT and CSF characteristics are thus those of BIH. This stresses the need to perform magnetic resonance imaging (MRI) and/or angiography systematically in all patients presenting with BIH. Thus, in a prospective series of 24 consecutive patients with BIH, angiography disclosed CVT in six (Tehindrazanarivelo *et al.*, 1992). Normal MRI and/or angiography should in our opinion be included in the diagnostic criteria of BIH.

FOCAL SIGNS

A second group of CVT is characterized by the presence of focal cerebral signs. This is the largest group, accounting for roughly 75% of published cases, but it is a heterogeneous one, depending on the mode of onset of symptoms, the nature of focal signs (deficits, seizures or both), and their possible association with signs of raised intracranial pressure and altered consciousness. Focal deficits of sudden onset – 23% in Ameri's series (1992) – simulate an arterial stroke, but the presence of seizures, the progression of symptoms and the absence of characteristic arterial distribution on the CT image should raise the possibility of CVT. Subacute cases with deficits or seizures – 25% in Ameri's series (1992) – point to a brain abscess or to viral encephalitis, and chronic cases (11%) to a tumour. Focal signs can be even more misleading when they present as transient ischaemic attacks (Bousser *et al.*, 1985) or migraine-like phenomena (Newman *et al.*, 1989).

CAVERNOUS SINUS SYNDROME

Cavernous sinus thrombosis has a distinctive clinical picture, which will be described later.

SUBACUTE ENCEPHALOPATHY

A fourth pattern of presentation is that of a subacute encephalopathy, i.e. a generalized encephalopathic illness without localizing signs or recognizable features of raised intracranial pressure. The patients are often either very old or very young, and suffering from cachexia, malignant or cardiac disease; the cerebral thrombosis may be a terminal event or even discovered by chance at autopsy (Barnett and Hyland, 1953). Dehydration and dysphagia are contributory causes in many cases, and there is a high prevalence of pulmonary embolism and venous thrombosis in other sites.

The location of vein or sinus occlusion in the brain is variable; it is often multiple, the unpaired sinuses (sagittal sinus, straight sinus) being most often involved. Clinical signs are non-localizing and a depressed level of consciousness is the most constant finding, varying from drowsiness to deep coma. Headache may be prominent but is often masked by drowsiness. Raised intracranial pressure is also difficult to detect and papilloedema may be absent. CSF pressure may be normal and the fluid may show evidence of slight haemorrhage or a mononuclear pleocytosis. Generalized seizures are common, especially in children, and attacks of trismus and decerebrate rigidity may also occur (Ehlers and Courville, 1936). Fever is generally absent and nuchal rigidity unusual. This type of presentation carries a high mortality and the brain at autopsy shows patchy or confluent neuronal damage with cortical laminar necrosis affecting cortical layers 3 and 5, and multiple haemorrhagic infarcts, either in cortex or basal ganglia (Towbin, 1973). The brain may show evidence of generalized swelling and tentorial herniation.

The diagnosis in this type of venous disease can be extremely difficult and the differential diagnosis includes encephalitis, disseminated intravascular coagulation, thrombotic thrombocytopenic purpura, marantic endocarditis, cerebral vasculitis and brain abscess. The occurrence of generalized cerebral symptoms, such as depressed conscious level or seizures even in the absence of raised intracranial pressure should raise the possibility of venous thrombosis. Provided that appropriate treatment to counter dehydration is given along with anticoagulation, the prognosis may not be as unfavourable as in the past.

OTHER PRESENTATIONS

The grouping of signs of CVT into these four main patterns (isolated intracranial hypertension (ICH), focal signs, cavernous sinus syndrome, subacute encephalopathy) does not account for every case. Some patients with isolated ICH later develop focal neurological signs (Bousser *et al.*, 1985; Feldenzer *et al.*, 1987; Einhäupl and Masuhr, 1994). Others present with headache of sudden onset, neck stiffness and CT scan, or lumbar puncture evidence of subarachnoid haemorrhage simulating a ruptured intracranial aneurysm (Bousser *et al.*, 1985). Isolated psychiatric disturbances such as delirium can be inaugural. They are particularly misleading when they occur post-partum, raising the possibility of post-partum psychosis (Ruel *et al.*, 1986). CVT can even be totally asymptomatic, as illustrated by one of the patients reported by Goldberg *et al.* (1986) who was found to have a left LS thrombosis without any symptom at a routine CT scan after mastoidectomy.

CLINICAL CHARACTERISTICS OF THROMBOSIS AT DEFINED SITES

DISTRIBUTION OF CEREBRAL VENOUS THROMBOSIS

The relative distribution of sites of CVT is indicated in Table 3.3. It should be considered as a rough estimate, particularly as far as cortical vein involvement is concerned, since it is often missed at angiography. Furthermore, it is uncommon for thrombosis to be confined to a single vessel. Thus in about 75% of cases, there is an involvement of multiple veins or sinuses (Bousser *et al.*, 1985; Ameri and Bousser, 1992; Cantu and Barinagarrementeria, 1993). In the majority of cases, thrombosis is an evolving process with propagation to adjacent vessels, but this might not be detected at angiography, which is usually performed only once.

The vessel most commonly affected is SSS: 72% in Ameri's series (1992), 85% in Daif's series (1995), 92% in Cantu's series (1992). It was involved alone in a minority of cases, respectively, 13%, 55% and 29% in the three series mentioned above. The LS is almost as often affected as SSS in some series – 70% for Ameri (1992) – but far less frequent in others (38%) (Cantu and Barinagarrementeria, 1993). Its isolated involvement is rare, respectively, 9% and 2%. Cerebral veins were affected in about 40% of cases (in Ameri's series) but this is probably an underestimation given the much higher frequency of focal clinical signs. Thrombosis of the Galenic system is rare, with some 60 reported cases. Only a

Table 3.3 Distribution of venous thrombosis in recent series of patients with CVT

Veins	Milandre *et al.* (1988)	Ameri and Bousser (1992)	Cantu and Barinagarrementeria (1993)		Tsai *et al.* (1995)	Daif *et al.* (1995)
			Puerperal	Non-puerperal		
	($n = 20$)	($n = 110$)	($n = 67$)	($n = 46$)	($n = 29$)	($n = 40$)
SSS	13 (4)	79 (14)	60 (22)	45 (11)	19 (11)	34 (22)
LS	2	78 (17)	23 (1)	20 (1)	15 (9)	14 (4)
SS	5	16 (1)	0	0	3	3
CS	1	3 (0)	0	0	0	
CV	10 (2)	45 (2)	13	14	1	4
DVS	1 (1)	9 (1)	17 (4)	10		
Association	12	75	39	34	9	26

Numbers in parentheses indicate cases in which the venous structure was involved alone.
SSS, superior sagittal sinus; LS, lateral sinus; SS, straight sinus; CS, cavernous sinus; CV, cortical or cerebellar veins; DVS, deep venous system.
Association: more than one structure involved.

few cases have been described of petrosal sinus, isolated cortical or cerebellar vein thrombosis, but these conditions are also likely to be underdiagnosed because of the extreme difficulty of their diagnosis.

The frequent multiple vein involvement, the variability of the cortical venous system, and the rapid development of collateral circulation explain the lack of well-defined topographic clinical syndromes similar to those described in arterial occlusion. There are, however, broad patterns according to the site of venous occlusion.

SUPERIOR SAGITTAL SINUS THROMBOSIS

SSS thrombosis is the most frequent form of CVT. It may occur from any of the causes discussed below, but its exposed position makes it a favoured site for traumatic thrombosis and for thrombosis secondary to meningeal infiltration. Its involvement is frequent in parasagittal meningioma and it is also the preferential site of puerperal CVT. Its clinical presentation is highly variable according to the involvement of adjacent cortical veins. When thrombosis is restricted to SSS, the clinical presentation is that of isolated ICH mimicking benign intracranial hypertension as described above. In Ameri's series (1992), 33% of 79 cases of SSS thrombosis presented as BIH. Grand-mal seizures and psychiatric disturbances occasionally occur in pure SSS thrombosis (Ruel *et al.*, 1986). In the majority of cases, thrombosis also involves one or both lateral sinus with again intracranial hypertension as the main clinical presentation. Extension to cortical veins, particularly the Rolandic and parietal veins, is frequent and is characterized by the acute or progressive onset of a focal motor or sensory deficit associated with focal or generalized seizures (see the description of Rolandic and parieto-occipital venous infarctions below). Some signs were classically considered as suggestive of SSS and adjacent cortical vein thrombosis such as a deficit more marked in the leg or a bilateral deficit. However, the bilateral or alternating deficits, which were considered as the hallmark of SSS thrombosis, now appear as rare and late features. They were encountered in only three patients in Ameri's series (1992).

The following four cases illustrate various patterns of presentation of SSS thrombosis.

A 26-year-old woman suffered from paroxysmal nocturnal haemoglobinuria since the age of 10. On 8 March 1995 she suddenly experienced bifrontal headache, which improved over the next few hours but recurred the next day, and became permanent within 5 days, associated with nausea and vomiting. A week later, she complained of blurred vision.

Examination revealed severe papilloedema with retinal haemorrhages and a macular involvement. Neurological examination was otherwise normal, as was a CT scan. MRI showed an increased SSS signal in T1- and T2-weighted imaging (WI) and magnetic resonance (MR) angiography did not visualize the SSS. CSF composition was normal but the pressure was increased (27 cm water). Heparin treatment was started immediately after lumbar puncture. The next day her headache started to improve and the blurring of vision disappeared within a few days.

This is a typical example of SSS thrombosis with isolated intracranial hypertension of subacute onset, in a young woman with paroxysmal nocturnal haemoglobinuria.

A 25-year-old woman was known to have cutaneous lupus. She had an uneventful pregnancy until the 30th week when she suddenly complained of severe abdominal pain with signs of acute fetal distress. A Caesarean section was immediately performed. The baby survived and the mother felt quite well. Three days later she suffered diffuse headache without other symptoms. Neurological examination and fundus were normal. Headache increased, and became permanent and lateralized on the right side. Two weeks after delivery, she sustained three Jacksonian seizures of the left arm and a grand-mal seizure. When she regained consciousness she had a dense left hemiplegia, more marked in the arm, without sensory or visual disturbances. CT scan without constrast showed a right-sided rolandic hyperdensity surrounded by a large hypodensity with a mass effect. MRI confirmed a large Rolandic haemorrhagic infarct and showed an increased SSS signal on T1- and T2-WI. Carotid angiography disclosed no injection of the anteror two thirds of the SSS and of adjacent rolandic veins. Anticonvulsants, steroids and heparin were given. The patient started to improve 24 hours after the onset of heparin and she recovered completely within 3 weeks.

This is a typical history of acute SSS and unilateral rolandic vein thrombosis with seizures and hemiplegia, but no obvious signs of ICH. The other interesting point is that heparin was given despite a haemorrhagic infarct, with a rapid and complete recovery.

A 62-year-old man was in excellent health until 20 November 1986 when he suddenly realized that he could no longer move his right foot. This lasted less than 1 minute and recovered completely. A few minutes later, the same paralysis recurred and lasted again about 30 seconds. The next morning, he suddenly was unable to move his right hand for a few minutes; he became aphasic and, at the same time, he experienced clonic movements of the left leg. The whole episode lasted 10 minutes and cleared completely, but later that day the patient experienced pins and needles in his right face for 2 minutes. Neurologic examination was entirely normal. CT scan without contrast was normal but showed an empty delta sign after injection. CSF was abnormal with increased protein (90 mg 100 ml^{-1}), increased lymphocytes (30 per mm^3), presence of red blood cells (5200). After CT scan, the patient had a focal seizure in the right leg. Angiography showed an occlusion of the middle third of SSS with non-injection of Rolandic and parietal veins. Heparin treatment was given, with a full recovery. No definite underlying cause for thrombosis was found except for infected teeth, which were treated with antibiotics.

This illustrates bilateral and alternating signs in SSS with bilateral cortical vein thrombosis. The other interesting points are: the acute onset; the mixture of transient focal deficits mimicking transient ishaemic attacks (TIAs) and focal seizures; and the absence of signs of raised intracranial pressure despite the bilateral involvement of cortical veins associated with SSS thrombosis.

A 36-year-old woman complained of headache, which worsened progressively over 2 weeks. She then started to experience transient visual obscurations. She was seen by an ophthalmologist who found bilateral papilloedema. She was advised to see a neurologist but the day before the appointment she suddenly complained of bilateral leg weakness. At examination she had an almost complete paraplegia with bilateral Babinski sign, and major disturbances of joint position and vibration sense. There were no abnormal findings in the arm and face. Brain CT scan disclosed a bilateral parasagittal hypodensity with patchy areas of increased density. Angiography disclosed an incomplete filling of SSS and an abrupt occlusion of the cortical veins in the parasagittal region (Figure 5.26, see page 114) Heparin treatment was immediately started and the patient made a full recovery. The only potential risk factor was the intake of oral contraceptives.

This is a case of SSS thrombosis with bilateral cortical vein thrombosis resulting in paraplegia and ICH

LATERAL SINUS THROMBOSIS

Thrombosis at this site may occur from any of the causes listed below, but it is particularly frequent as a consequence of acute or chronic ear and mastoid infection. Southwick *et al.* (1986) found 64 cases of septic LS thrombosis fully reported between 1940 and 1984.

Like SSS thrombosis, LS thrombosis has a variable presentation, according to the extent of the thrombotic process. Although it can be asymptomatic, isolated LS thrombosis usually manifests as raised intracranial pressure, hence the term of 'otitic hydrocephalus' coined by Symonds (1956) to describe the effect of LS thrombosis secondary to an active or latent ear infection. The classical picture is that of a child who, a variable time after otitis, may experience continuing earache and fever, associated with neck pain and headache. Pain and tenderness may be present along the anterior border of the sternomastoid muscle, in the mastoid region (Hawkins, 1985). Headache increases rapidly and in 3–15 days, and other signs of intracranial hypertension develop. As already mentioned, LS thrombosis is rarely isolated and more frequently extends to other sinuses and veins, especially to the SSS presenting as isolated intracranial hypertension. Thus the majority of patients with LS thrombosis do not have focal signs. These occur when thrombosis extends to superior or inferior petrosal sinuses with respectively fifth and sixth cranial nerve involvement, to the straight sinus and deep venous system (see below), to adjacent cortical veins with aphasia in left LS thrombosis (see below), and to the jugular bulb with involvement of the ninth, tenth and eleventh cranial nerves.

The following case reports illustrate two main presentations of LS thrombosis: isolated ICH and dysphasia owing to an associated posterior temporal venous infarction. The third is a most unusual case of subarachnoid haemorrhage owing to a lateral and straight sinus thrombosis.

A 39-year-old woman complained of headache in January 1994. This was initially frontal, but rapidly became diffuse and severe. Three weeks later she experienced transient visual obscurations when coughing and stooping. She also noticed horizontal diplopia on extreme lateral gaze on both sides. At examination, there was a severe papilloedema with peripapillary haemorrhages. Neurologic examination was otherwise normal. CSF composition was normal but pressure increased (27 cm water). MRI showed on T1- and T2-images an increased signal of the whole right lateral sinus. Erythrocyte sedimentation rate (ESR) was increased (57 mm), white blood cell (WBC) count was 13 000. There was a past history of deep vein thrombosis in 1993. Genital and buccal aphthous ulcers appeared while she was in hospital. Behçet's disease was diagnosed.

This is a typical presentation of intracranial hypertension in an isolated right lateral sinus thrombosis.

In 1982, a 32-year-old woman had an uneventful second pregnancy when she suddenly sustained a series of epileptic seizures, which lasted 3 days after which she remained comatose for 2 days. When the coma resolved the only abnormal clinical signs were a moderate predominantly motor dysphasia without alexia and agraphia, and a mild right-sided facial weakness. CT scan showed a left temporal hypodensity and angiography disclosed a left lateral sinus thrombosis, and a thrombosis of the vein of Labbé. She was treated with anticonvulsants and heparin. Within 5 days, all symptoms disappeared. Her pregnancy continued normally and delivery was normal. Six months later, despite anticonvulsants, she suffered partial complex seizures with the very strange feeling that she was again doing what she had done in the previous hours, but in the reverse order and at a very high speed 'as a film going backwards'. Further investigations were performed and she was found to have systemic lupus.

This is a left sinus thrombosis, which, in itself, was silent, but was associated with a thrombosis of the vein of Labbé responsible for a temporal lobe infarct. This manifested with status epilepticus and a mild focal deficit. Another interesting point concerns the aetiology: CVT was thought to be pregnancy related until late recurrent seizures led to the discovery of systemic lupus.

A 22-year-old Algerian woman was perfectly well when, on 1 May 1987, she suddenly experienced an excruciating headache. CT scan and lumbar puncture showed a subarachnoid haemorrhage. Carotid angiography was normal. The patient improved but 4 days later the same explosive headache recurred. She was transferred to a neurosurgical department in Paris where the diagnosis of subarachnoid haemorrhage was confirmed. A four-vessel angiography showed no vascular malformation, but disclosed thrombosis of the left lateral sinus and of straight sinus. No treatment was given and the patient made an uneventful recovery.

This is a rare case of sinus thrombosis with subarachnoid haemorrhage as the only manifestation. The thrombosis involved the lateral sinus and straight sinus without involvement of the SSS, which is also an unusual combination.

CORTICAL VEIN THROMBOSIS

Any cortical vein can be the seat of thrombosis but those most often involved are the superior cerebral veins that drain into the SSS. It is suggested that the primary site of thrombosis is at the junction of cortical vein and superior sagittal sinus or in the lacunae. Mural thrombus enlarges until it blocks the cortical vein and then propagates backwards as a red thrombus in the stagnant stream towards the pial plexus. Thrombus may also propagate in an anterograde direction along the sinus as an elongated grey tongue of fibrin/platelet thrombus without blocking the sinus. The consequences of a cortical vein thrombosis are variable; in an unknown proportion of cases, collateral circulation rapidly develops and there is no parenchymal lesion. In other cases, an area of localized oedema appears, which can still be asymptomatic. At a further stage, neurones become oedematous or partially ischaemic, but this injury is mostly reversible as judged by the frequency of totally regressive focal deficits. Even when an infarct occurs, confirmed at neuro-imaging, it is remarkable that clinical recovery can still in some cases be complete.

The amount of infarction is variable, depending on the extent of thrombosis and the availability of venous collateral pathways. Isolated cortical vein thrombosis was classically thought to be relatively common: Garcin and Pestel (1949) in their review of 57 published cases of CVT found 15 cases (26%) but this high frequency is probably the result of a diagnostic bias: many of these cases were mistaken for an abscess or a tumour and were operated on. The diagnosis of CVT was established at surgery whereas in most other forms of CVT, the *intra vitam* diagnosis was not possible and CVT was discovered only at autopsy. More recently, in their review of the neuropathology of CVT, Cervos-Navarro and Kannuki (1990) found isolated thrombosis of cortical veins in 6% of cases. In the recent literature based on neuroimaging, well-documented cases are extremely rare, with an overall frequency of about 2% in the two largest series (Ameri and Bousser, 1992; Cantu and Barinagarrementeria, 1993). In the majority of cases, thrombosis of cortical veins extend to SSS [21% in Cantu's series (1993), 35% in Ameri's series (1992)] and occasionally to cortical veins on the opposite side, leading to the classical picture of a bilateral and often haemorrhagic infarct, with cortical and subcortical necrosis maximal in the parasagittal region.

Although venous infarction can affect any region of the brain and although there are no defined venous territories corresponding to those of the major cerebral arteries, there are some locations that tend to be more frequently affected. These are usually situated in the posterior part of the hemispheres and adjacent to SSS or LS, affecting the Rolandic, parieto-occipital and posterior temporal regions. The clinical counterpart of these cortical infarcts is the presence of focal deficits and/or seizures, but their pattern differs according to the site of the lesion.

Rolandic venous infarction

This is the result of thrombosis of the superficial cortical veins, which drain the pre- and post-central gyri and join the SSS, which is frequently involved. It extends for a variable distance over the lateral surface of the posterior frontal and anterior parietal lobes on each side of the central sulcus. It produces a characteristic clinical picture well described by Holmes and Sargent (1915) in traumatic sagittal sinus thrombosis, and by Martin and Sheehan (1941) in puerperal cases. There is hemiparesis, unilateral or bilateral, affecting the leg more than the arm and usually sparing the face. Speech is seldom impaired. The appearance of the hemiparesis is often abrupt, suggesting an arterial stroke, and it frequently follows a focal seizure. On other occasions hemiparesis may be transient or repetitive, disappearing in a few minutes or hours. Sometimes the symptoms may alternate from side to side. In the affected leg weakness is more pronounced in the distal than the proximal part and an unusual type of hypertonus described as plastic rigidity is an early feature. Cortical sensory loss with marked astereognosis is present and is again more obvious in the lower limb. If the Rolandic vein is thrombosed at some distance from the sagittal sinus, the weakness may involve the arm and face more than leg. Cortical sensory loss is again a prominent finding. A cramp-like contracture of the hand was described by Martin and Sheehan (1941). Focal epilepsy, which may proceed to generalized attacks, frequently involves the whole of one side and may be followed by a post-ictal paralysis. Very localized attacks affecting only the upper face have been recorded (Dowman, 1926). Repeated or continuous focal seizures are a particular feature of cortical venous infarction in this region.

Parieto-occipital venous infarction

This is the result of thrombosis of the parietal group of superficial cortical veins that join the SSS in its posterior third. It is centred on the parieto-occipital sulcus extending for a variable distance laterally towards the angular gyrus. It may be unilateral or bilateral, and SSS is most frequently involved. It affects those regions of the brain concerned with the orientation and spatial characterization of visual stimuli, with object recognition and with oculomotor pursuit movements. Damage to this area, particularly if bilateral, produces the syndrome of visual disorientation where the patient has difficulty in the judgement of distance and in visually guided movements, in gauging the relative size of objects and in counting numbers of objects. In addition there is defective smooth pursuit and refixation eye movement (psychic paralysis of gaze), absence of blinking reaction to a visual threat (Balint's syndrome) (Martin, 1944). Amnesia, anosagnosia and hallucinosis have also been recorded (Sakurai *et al.*, 1992). If the infarct is extensive, it may involve the upper fibres of the visual radiation causing a lower altitudinal hemianopia. However, dense and complete homonymous hemianopia occurs extremely rarely. Seizures may be present but are not so frequent as in more anteriorly situated infarction.

A man with thrombosis of the superior sagittal sinus presenting with bilateral parieto-occipital infarction and raised intracranial pressure

A 61-year-old man complained of severe neck pain following a neck manipulation followed a few days later by blurring of vision, difficulty with reading and in using his right arm. He was a heavy cigarette smoker with intermittent claudication and with absent pulses below the knees. Examination showed a confused and drowsy patient with a right hemiparesis and right lower quadrant anopia. The left visual field was also abnormal with defective visual localization and visual inattention, worse in the lower quadrant. He had dyslexia, dyscalculia and finger agnosia. There was early swelling of both optic discs and a right sixth nerve palsy.

A CT scan showed a patchy bilateral occipito-parietal haemorrhagic infarction with oedema, worse on the left side, and further smaller regions of infarction in both frontal lobes and in the left cerebellar hemisphere.

Spinal fluid was under greatly increased pressure (45 cm) with normal constituents. MR angiography showed thrombotic occlusion of the superior sagittal sinus in its posterior third. The left lateral sinus was also thrombosed. A full haematological examination showed no prothrombotic abnormality and there was no sign of systemic disease.

The patient improved following treatment of cerebral swelling with dexamethasone but developed further visual loss secondary to papilloedema, which required bilateral optic nerve-sheath fenestration. Anticoagulant treatment was recommended but declined. He eventually made a good recovery apart from impaired visual acuity from secondary optic atrophy.

Posterior temporal venous infarction

This is situated more inferiorly. It is almost always unilateral and follows thrombosis of the inferior anastomotic vein (Labbé) or one of the inferior middle cerebral veins draining downwards into the lateral sinus. Infarcts in this region tend to produce a contralateral hemiparesis of brachio-facial type with cortical sensory loss and rarely homonymous hemianopia. Focal and generalized seizures may occur (Dorndorf *et al.*, 1993). In the dominant hemisphere there may be an amnestic type of dysphasia with alexia, agraphia, acalculia and finger agnosia. Isolated thrombosis of the vein of Labbé has been reported only in a few cases: there was a lobar subcortical haemorrhagic infarct in all cases and the main sign was aphasia; it was of the sensory type in two cases (Kawase *et al.*, 1983; Komiyama *et al.*, 1988) and of the motor type in another one (Cambria, 1980). A remarkable case has been reported by Yokota *et al.* (1990) of a pure agraphia of Kanji (the Japanese morphograms) contrasting with a preservation of writing Kana (the Japanese syllabograms), and of reading both Kanji and Kana. There was no aphasia, apraxia or disturbance of consciousness.

In conclusion, the clinical presentation of cortical vein thrombosis remains poorly known because isolated cortical vein thrombosis is both rare and difficult to diagnose. Furthermore, most accounts fail to distinguish between the features of cortical vein thrombosis and sinus thrombosis. The hallmark of cortical vein thrombosis is a focal hemispheric deficit, seizure, or both, commonly of sudden onset, but occasionally with a steady or stepwise progression mimicking a space occupying lesion. In most cases however, there is extension to SSS with signs of raised intracranial pressure as described above. The following case is one of the few documented examples of isolated cortical vein thrombosis.

A 74-year-old man had a past history of atrial fibrillation with a deep right middle cerebral artery infarct in 1980. He had been taking oral anticoagulants since then. In 1988, a prostatic carcinoma was discovered and surgically treated. On 22 May 1988 he had a fall with a huge leg haematoma. Anticoagulants were discontinued but 3 days later he had a grand-mal seizure with a right post-ictal hemiplegia, which recovered in 15 minutes. At neurologic examination, there was a very mild left hemiparesis, which was thought to be the sequel of the 1980 stroke. A CT scan without contrast showed a punctiform spontaneous hyperdensity in the left Rolandic region. MRI disclosed, on T2-WI images, an increased signal in the right deep MCA territory (sequelae of the 1980 stroke) and a spontaneous hypersignal of a cortical vein on the left side (Figure 5:46 see page 130). Left carotid angiography showed normal sinuses but absent Rolandic veins replaced by multiple collateral dilated 'corkscrew' vessels. Anticoagulant treatment was resumed and no further event occurred.

This is a Rolandic vein thrombosis manifesting only with a grand-mal seizure and a 15 minutes post-ictal hemiplegia. CT and MRI abnormalities were minimal but angiography was typical of cortical vein thrombosis. This illustrates how such a diagnosis can be difficult. The onset of seizure 3 days after stopping anticoagulants was suggestive of CVT.

THROMBOSIS OF THE DEEP VENOUS SYSTEM (GALENIC SYSTEM)

Thrombosis of the Galenic system is much less common than SSS or LS thrombosis with some 60 detailed reported cases. In their review of 57 reported clinicopathological cases of CVT, Garcin and Pestel (1949) found ten cases of thrombosis of the Galenic system. The proportion was 8% in Ameri's series (1992) and 24% in the Mexican series (Cantu and Barinagarrementeria, 1993). It is sometimes associated with sinus thrombosis in a widespread and almost always fatal intracerebral venous thrombotic disease (Ehlers and Courville, 1936; Huhn, 1965). Isolated Galenic system thrombosis has been reported mostly in children. Its extent is variable: most often the whole of the Galenic system with its large tributaries (basal veins of Rosenthal, internal cerebral veins, great vein of Galen and straight sinus) is involved. A bilateral haemorrhagic infarct is observed affecting the corpus striatum, septum pellucidum, thalamus, hypothalamus, the ventral corpus callosum, the medial occipital lobe and the superior surface of the cerebellum (Figure 2.3). There is intense congestion of the choroid plexus and often intraventricular haemorrhage (Ehlers and Courville, 1936; Garcin and Pestel, 1949; Bots, 1971; Johnsen *et al.*, 1973; Eick *et al.*, 1981; Ur Rahman and Al-Tahan, 1993). In some cases, however, there is a limited involvement of the major veins, such as internal cerebral veins and basal veins, or of small veins, such as the choroidal, thalamo-striate or anterior cerebral veins. In Ameri's series there was only one case of thrombosis limited to one of the major veins: a case of bilateral thrombosis of the basal vein of Rosenthal. Isolated involvement of straight sinus is extremely rare. It is usually associated either with thrombosis of the vein of Galen or with thrombosis of superficial sinuses: SSS, lateral sinuses or both.

The clinical presentation is highly variable. The classic picture of extensive Galenic system thrombosis is that of a child with an acute coma associated with decerebration, decortication, extrapyramidal hypertonus, signs of raised intracranial pressure, pupillary changes and rise in blood pressure leading to death in a few hours or, more commonly, in a few days (Ehlers and Courville, 1936; Johnsen *et al.*, 1973; Eick *et al.*, 1981). Similar cases have been reported in adults. One of the first cases was described by Garcin and Pestel (1947) during the puerperium. It was characterized by severe headaches followed 2 days later by coma, left hemiparesis and hyperthermia, which led to death in less than 48 hours. Autopsy showed an isolated thrombosis of the deep venous system. Another case has been recently been reported in a young woman who presented with a 3 months history of isolated ICH owing to an undiagnosed sinus thrombosis. She was admitted because of obtundation and sudden worsening of headache. Within 24 hours she became deeply comatose with bilateral extensor plantar responses, episodic decerebrate posturing and

Cheyne–Stokes respiration. She died a few hours later. CT scan showed an extensive thrombosis of the deep venous system (Ur Rahman and Al-Tahan, 1993) (Figures 5.17, 5.18, see pages 104 and 105). When patients survive, severe sequelae are frequent, such as akinetic mutism, mental retardation, dementia, bilateral athetoid movements, hemiparesis, vertical gaze palsy and dystonia (Ehlers and Courville, 1936; Garcin and Pestel, 1947, 1949; Bots, 1971; Solomon *et al.*, 1982). In Ameri's series of nine patients, sequelae were observed in three. The following report is that of the most severely affected of these patients.

A 32-year-old Algerian man with known Behçet's disease complained in June 1983 of headache, which rapidly worsened and was associated with memory disturbances and disorientation. He also complained of visual disturbances and difficulties in swallowing. When he was examined 2 months later, he was bedridden with upward vertical gaze palsy, bilateral facial weakness, pseudobulbar palsy, bilateral grasping, right hemiparesis, sphincter incontinence and dementia of the subcortical type. A CSF study showed a normal protein content but increased lymphocytes (12 per mm^3). A CT scan showed a bilateral diencephalic hypodensity (Figure 5.10, see page 98) and angiography disclosed thrombosis of internal cerebral and basal veins. Heparin and steroid treatment were started; an indisputable improvement was observed, but memory disturbances and abulia persisted.

This is a severe case of subacute isolated thrombosis of the basal veins of Rosenthal, in the course of a known Behçet's disease, with neuropsychological sequelae.

Recent reports have illustrated the possibility of benign forms of Galenic system thrombosis. These forms have probably been underestimated in the past because the deep venous system was frequently not visualized at conventional angiography owing to the delay in emptying when there was a massive cerebral oedema. Such benign forms were encountered in six out of nine cases in Ameri's series. The clinical features are often ill defined; the most regular symptoms are headache, nausea and vomiting, gait ataxia, neuropsychological deficits and drowsiness of a variable degree [Johnsen *et al.*, 1973 (case 2); Eick *et al.*, 1981 (case 3); Chilvers and Rudge, 1986; Kim and Walczak, 1986; Haley *et al.*, 1989; Baumgartner and Landis, 1992]. Other signs are unusual and include impaired upward conjugate gaze, vertical nystagmus, hemiparesis, which may be bilateral or alternating, limb or axial rigidity, tremor, seizures and signs of raised intracranial pressure. Neuropsychological disturbances are constant, although they can be transiently masked by impaired consciousness. Baumgartner and Landis (1992) in their review of seven patients who survived a venous thalamic infarction found that all had an impaired anterograde memory and that those with left-sided thalamic infarctions were dysphasic, irrespective of additional lenticulocapsular involvement. A severe amnesic syndrome with confabulation resembling Korsakoff's psychosis has been documented by Haley *et al.* (1989), in a 18-year-old female who also exhibited disorientation, abulia, attentional deficits, dyscalculia and impaired IQ scores. In that case and in the seven others collected by Baumgartner and Landis (1992), clinical outcome was good with either no sequelae or a very mild residual memory impairment. The diagnosis of these benign forms of Galenic system thrombosis is particularly difficult because of the variability and lack of specificity of the clinical presentation. Suspicion should be raised when CT scan shows a bilateral lesion, usually hypodense, but occasionally with some hyperdense patches, involving basal ganglia and the surrounding white matter. One of our patients illustrates the neuropsychological presentation and benign outcome of some bilateral deep venous system thrombosis.

> A 37-year-old woman had no past history but started to suffer headaches in May 1976. This progressively worsened, and the patient became apathetic and occasionally disoriented. At examination in August 1976 there was apathy, abulia, disorientation, a severe amnesic syndrome and a mild left hemiparesis. Electroencephalogram (EEG) showed a right-sided slow activity, CSF disclosed pleocytosis (25 lymphocytes mm^{-3}); isotope brain scanning with technetium-99m was normal, carotid angiography was considered as normal (CT was not yet available). No diagnosis was established and a complete recovery occurred spontaneously in September 1976. A year later (August 1977), headache recurred with nausea, vomiting and papilloedema, in a context of fever, raised sedimentation rate and aphthous ulcers. Carotid angiography disclosed SSS thrombosis and the diagnosis of Behçet's disease was established. In the light of the diagnosis, the angiogram performed the year before was re-examined and it was obvious that there was an extensive thrombosis of the internal cerebral veins, vein of Galen and straight sinus. Figure 5.25 see page 114).

The clinical signs of this patient are typical of benign deep venous system thrombosis with an insidious onset and a spontaneous recovery. It is also an illustration of CVT as first sign of Behçet's disease.

CEREBELLAR VEIN THROMBOSIS

Cerebellar venous infarction is extremely rare and until recently it was not recognized during life (Noetzel and Jerusalem, 1965). It usually affects the cerebellar hemisphere and may follow thrombosis of some of the surface veins draining into the transverse or petrosal sinuses, or of the superior vermian vein, which drains into the vein of Galen. Isolated cerebellar vein thrombosis has not been reported and in all published cases there was an associated sinus thrombosis, mainly lateral sinuses (Stevens and Ammerman, 1959; Bousser *et al.*, 1985; Rousseaux *et al.*, 1988; Nayak *et al.*, 1994), straight sinus (Bousser *et al.*, 1985; Eng *et al.*, 1990) or even multiple sinuses (Bousser *et al.*, 1985; Chilvers and Rudge, 1986). As usual in CVT, the corresponding infarct can be haemorrhagic, unilateral or bilateral, and it is usually surrounded by oedema. Because of the limited volume of the posterior fossa, there is early obstruction of CSF circulation with resultant hydrocephalus (Averback, 1978; Rousseaux *et al.*, 1988). Upward and downward herniation of the cerebellum, and fatal brainstem compression may occur unless the pressure is relieved.

The clinical presentation is variable. The most frequent signs are headache, vomiting and ataxia. They are usually of acute onset but subacute (Rousseaux *et al.*, 1988) and even chronic cases (Bousser *et al.*, 1985) have been reported. There is an early decrease in conscious level and frequent papilloedema indicating obstructive hydrocephalus. The combination of unilateral cerebellar dysmetria with headache and signs of raised intracranial pressure is suggestive of cerebellar infarction (Rousseaux *et al.*, 1988; Nayak *et al.*, 1994). There is usually no marked hemiparesis, but the limbs may show bilateral brisk reflexes and extensor plantar responses. Generalized seizures may occur signifying either acute hydrocephalus, or the spread of thrombosis to SSS and adjacent cortical veins. Cranial nerve palsies can occur (Boussser *et al.*, 1985) and the involvement of the ninth and tenth nerves may suggest propagation of thrombosis to the internal jugular vein (Symonds, 1956). Brain CT scan invariably shows hydrocephalus, whereas the aspect of the cerebellum is variable: normal in some cases, showing a hypodense mass lesion with contrast enhancement in others (Bousser *et al.*, 1985; Rousseaux *et al.*, 1988), and showing a unilateral or bilateral haemorrhage in others (Eng *et al.*, 1990).

The outcome is variable: among recent reports, a complete recovery was observed in three cases (Stevens and Ammerman, 1959; Bousser *et al.*, 1985; Nayak *et al.*, 1994), sequelae were observed in two cases (Bousser *et al.*, 1985; Rousseaux *et al.*, 1988) and death occurred in two patients (Chilvers and Rudge, 1986; Eng *et al.*, 1990). As in arterial cerebellar infarcts, surgery is required in some patients with life-threatening hydrocephalus, to insert a shunt or to remove the swollen cerebellar infarct (Stevens and Ammerman, 1959; Rousseaux *et al.*, 1988). There is no aetiological specificity of cerebellar venous thrombosis: reported causes are chronic suppurative otitis media (Nayak *et al.*, 1944), oral contraceptive use (Chilvers and Rudge, 1986), pregnancy (Stevens and Ammerman, 1959), antithrombin deficiency (Bousser *et al.*, 1985) and in other cases no cause was found (Bousser *et al.*, 1985; Rousseaux *et al.*, 1988). The following observations are illustrative of two different forms of cerebellar vein thrombosis.

A 42-year-old woman was in excellent health until December 1980 when she first experienced episodes of vertigo and dizziness, which worsened rapidly and were associated with vomiting, gait instability, diplopia and difficulty in swallowing. At examination in March 1981, there were multiple cranial nerve palsies involving all nerves from the fifth to the eleventh of the left side, bilateral papilloedema and a left cerebellar incoordination. CT scan showed a spontaneous hyperdensity at the posterior part of the third ventricle with hydrocephalus. A ventriculo-atrial shunt was inserted on 4 April. Ventricular CSF contained 17 lymphotytes mm^3, 143 red bloods cells and increased protein 147 mg 100 ml^{-1}. Over the next 3 weeks the patient improved considerably with disappearance of headache and diplopia. A control CT scan without contrast was normal. However from 3 to 15 May, she had four transient ischaemic attacks, two with left-hand anaesthesia, one with left cheiro-oral paraesthesiae, one with right facial weakness. A four-vessel angiogram was performed, which showed an occlusion of the middle third of the SSS, the cortical parietal veins and the left vermian vein. There was also an incomplete and irregular filling of the left lateral sinus. Only then was the diagnosis of CVT established. She was treated with heparin and sustained an important improvement but with a mild left incoordination and a partial left seventh nerve palsy as sequelae. No cause was found despite extensive investigations.

In summary this case is remarkable for the following reasons:

1. It is a chronic case of cerebellar vein thrombosis with hydrocephalus, which mimicked a posterior fossa tumour.
2. The cerebellar vein thrombosis progressively extended to the lateral sinus, SSS and cortical veins.

3. The cortical vein thrombosis was characterized by transient focal deficits typical of transient ischaemic attacks.
4. The prognosis was good despite the extensive involvement of sinuses and veins.
5. No cause was found despite repeated investigation during the 16 years following.

A 46-year-old man suddenly complained of diffuse and severe headache without any other symptom. Fundus and neurological examination were normal, but there was a deep vein thrombosis of the left leg. CT scan showed a left cerebellar hypodensity with contrast enhancement. Four-vessel angiography disclosed occlusion of the left LS and of the left superior vermian vein. Antithrombin deficiency was discovered. Headache resolved in a week with heparin treatment.

This case illustrates a mild form of cerebellar vein thrombosis, with a sudden headache as the only sign (Sauron *et al.*, 1982).

CAVERNOUS SINUS THROMBOSIS

The cavernous sinus receives its main venous inflow from the face and orbit via the superior and inferior ophthalmic veins and the angular vein. Some of the superficial cerebral veins also drain into the sinus and thrombosis may spread from the sinus to the brain by this route. The outflow from the cavernous sinus is to the transverse sinus by the superior petrosal sinus and to the jugular bulb by the inferior petrosal sinus. There are important connections via emissary veins to the pterygoid plexus and the sphenoid sinus. The oculomotor and trochlear cranial nerves, along with the ophthalmic and maxillary branches of the trigeminal nerve course along the lateral wall of the cavernous sinus. Within the centre of the sinus itself are contained the abducens nerve and the carotid artery with its surrounding sympathetic neural plexus (Figure 1.10). This anatomical situation explains that oculomotor disturbances are almost invariably present in cavernous sinus thrombosis.

Cavernous sinus thrombosis used to be frequent and extremely severe: Grove (1936) was able to collect 400 cases and noted that the mortality was practically 100%. Since the introduction of antibiotics, cases are now reported less frequently and the prognosis has improved. It is, however, still a feared complication of sepsis in the nose or orbit (anterior route of propagation of infection), less commonly in the paranasal sinuses and teeth (inferior route), or in the middle ear (posterior route via the petrosal sinuses). The majority of cases are still infective in origin, with *Staphylococcus aureus* as the most frequent infecting organism, incriminated in over two-thirds of cases (Southwick *et al.*, 1986; DiNubile, 1988). Pneumococci and other streptococcal species account for the majority of the remaining cases; gram-negative bacilli, anaerobic bacteria and fungal infections, such as *Aspergillus fumigatus* (Sekhar *et al.*, 1980), also occur. In many cases the infective organism is not found (Clifford Jones *et al.*, 1982). Non-infective causes include head trauma, surgery, prothrombotic states (Melamed *et al.*, 1976) and dural arteriovenous malformation, either in the neighbourhood of the cavernous sinus or at a more distant site in the anterior part of the brain.

The clinical features of septic cavernous sinus thrombosis result from a combination of facial or upper respiratory tract cellulitis and obstruction of the sinus. In classic acute cases, there is an almost universal triad of chemosis proptosis and painful ophthalmoplegia, initially unilateral but frequently becoming bilateral (Garcin and Pestel, 1949; Coquillat and Warter, 1976; Clifford-Jones *et al.*, 1982; Gates, 1986; Southwick *et al.*, 1986; DiNubile, 1988; Levine *et al.*, 1988).

The first symptom is usually headache and facial pain, and the first indication that the sinus is involved is oedema and redness of the face, eyelid and conjunctiva accompanied by a worsening of fever and slight proptosis. This is followed by ophthalmoplegia (first the sixth nerve followed by the third and fourth) with further proptosis, papilloedema, and orbital and retinal congestion from obstruction of the superior and inferior orbital veins and the retinal veins. Pupillary reactions may be preserved in spite of an oculomotor palsy. Visual loss may occur from corneal ulceration, ischaemic optic neuropathy, central retinal artery occlusion or carotid arteritis. Facial sensory disturbances with pain and sensory loss are often overlooked, but are found in the majority of cases and indicate involvement of the ophthalmic and maxillary divisions of the trigeminal nerve (Southwick *et al.*, 1986). In severe cases there may be meningeal irritation or frank meningitis producing headache, vomiting and decreased conscious level. The internal carotid artery, which passes through the cavernous sinus, may be involved in the infection producing a focal arteritis with narrowing or occlusion on angiography (Matthew *et al.*, 1971; Segall *et al.*, 1982; Curnes *et al.*, 1987). The formation of a carotido-cavernous fistula has been recorded (Morvas and Morvas, 1968). Arterial embolism of infected thrombus may result in mycotic aneurysms (Micheli *et al.*, 1989) or multiple cerebral infarcts (Weisman, 1944; Kaplan and Mickle, 1984). A few cases have been reported of acute pituitary necrosis complicating cavernous sinus thrombosis (Weisman, 1944) and also of progressive hypopituitarism in the months following the thrombosis (Ivey and Smith, 1968).

The acute onset of chemosis, proptosis and painful ophthalmoplegia in the context of infection of the face is immediately suggestive of cavernous sinus thrombosis, but it is not specific and can also be encountered in orbital cellulitis, rhinocerebral mucormycosis and carotico-cavernous fistula. CT scanning, MRI and eventually angiography will establish the diagnosis (DiNubile, 1988).

A very similar presentation can also be observed in dural arterio-venous fistulae with thrombosis of ophthalmic veins as illustrated by the following case.

A 9-year-old Asian boy presented with a 6-week history of pain, diplopia and proptosis of the left eye. There was a history of febrile convulsions and a facial palsy when aged 3. Examination showed a 3 mm proptosis with some downward displacement of the left eye. There was no chemosis but retinal veins were engorged. Visual acuity and fields were normal. There was slight left ptosis and limitation of upward gaze in the left eye with vertical diplopia. Lateral movements and pupils were normal. A loud continuous bruit with systolic accentuation was heard over both orbits. Angiography showed a large dural arteriovenous malformation adjacent to the SSS in the frontal region at some distance from the cavernous sinus. It was fed by dural, ophthalmic and intracerebral arteries, and drained mainly into the sagittal sinus. A mass in the left orbit, above and medial to the globe indicated a thrombosed superior ophthalmic vein. No treatment was given and the proptosis and ophthalmoplegia gradually subsided; bruits persisted over both orbits.

Cavernous sinus thrombosis is not always acute but can also take a more indolent form, either spontaneously or because of the masking effect of an inadequate antibiotic regimen. The orbital manifestations are often unimpressive and an isolated sixth nerve palsy is the most consistent early neurologic sign, often associated with a mild headache. Chemosis and proptosis can be very moderate. A spontaneous improvement can even occur as in the remarkable case reported by Barraquer-Bordas *et al.* in 1955.

A 44-year-old man without any history of infection insidiously developed a mild left orbital pain followed some days later by horizontal diplopia, numbness of the left half of the forehead and a slight ptosis. These signs worsened over 2 months and disappeared over 2–3 months. The pain recurred with decreased visual acuity in the left eye leading to investigations and demonstration of left cavernous sinus thrombosis 7 months after the onset of symptoms. A complete recovery was observed after antibiotic and heparin treatment. Such subacute and chronic cases lead to great diagnostic difficulties and are sometimes mistaken for the Tolosa–Hunt syndrome (DiNubile, 1988).

The prognosis of cavernous sinus thrombosis has been considerably improved since the introduction of antibiotics. Yarrington (1977) estimated that the mortality had dropped to 12–14% but, in his review, DiNubile (1988) stated that the mortality rate was still approximately 30% and that less than half the patients recover completely. Others are left with various sequelae, most frequently visual: sixth nerve palsy, decreased visual acuity with optic atrophy and signs of aberrant regeneration of the third nerve (Brown, 1961).

THROMBOSIS OF PETROSAL SINUSES

Thrombosis of the superior and inferior petrosal sinuses is usually a sequel of cavernous sinus thrombosis or of infection in the temporal bone. Symonds (1956) pointed out the frequency of sixth nerve palsy in otitic hydrocephalus and suggested that the cause is spread of thrombosis from the lateral to the inferior petrosal sinus. These two structures are adjacent to one another at the petrous apex in Dorello's canal. He also observed occasional examples of the jugular foramen syndrome (paralysis of the ninth, tenth and eleventh cranial nerves) following thrombosis of the lateral sinus and internal jugular vein in patients with severe tonsillar infection or otitis media. Thrombosis of the superior petrosal sinus may induce facial and ear pain by involvement of the trigeminal nerve (Garcin and Pestel, 1949).

JUGULAR VEIN THROMBOSIS

Thrombosis may begin in the internal jugular vein or may spread there from the sigmoid sinus. In either case the commonest causes are infective, derived from otitic infection in the temporal bone or by spread from the oro-pharynx (Lemierre syndrome). Pharyngeal infections may be caused by streptococci, proteus, anaerobic or unusual organisms, such as *Fusobacterium necrophorum* (Ieven *et al.*, 1993). An increasing cause in recent times has been jugular vein thrombosis initiated by cannulae used for long-term venous access for drugs or parenteral nutrition, particularly in patients with malignant disease (Stephens *et al.*, 1991; Keidan, 1993). There are isolated reports of internal jugular thrombosis in association with polycythaemia vera (Guijarro *et al.*, 1995), carcinoma of the thyroid (Raveh *et al.*, 1995) and leiomyosarcoma of the omentum (Saponaro *et al.*, 1994). Obstruction to flow in the jugular vein leading to thrombosis may occur with metastatic deposits in the base of skull or from lesions such as a glomus jugulare tumour. Thrombosis may follow surgical dissection of neck glands and rarely carotid endarterectomy.

Internal jugular vein thrombosis has some special clinical features. There may be obvious signs of local infection with pain and swelling in the mastoid region and the tender thrombosed vein may be palpable. Torticollis may result from spasm of the adjacent sternomastoid muscle. A jugular foramen syndrome (paralysis of the ninth and tenth cranial nerves) may be present if the infection involves the skull base. Alteration in consciousness level owing to acutely raised intracranial pressure may occur when the neck is rotated.

The risk of venous thromboembolism to the lungs appears to be greater in jugular than in intracranial thrombosis and, in rare instances, there may be widespread propagation of thrombus to the superior vena cava and subclavian veins (Finn *et al.*, 1993). Intracranial retrograde propagation into the lateral sinus is indicated by signs of intracranial hypertension and is more likely to occur on the right side. The diagnosis is made by contrast venography but has been much simplified recently by the introduction of MRA and Döppler ultrasound (Finn *et al.*, 1993). Treatment of jugular thrombosis consists of anticoagulant or sometimes thrombolytic therapy combined with medical and surgical attention to the underlying cause, usually infective. The prognosis of deep-seated neck infections and necrotizing fasciitis, formerly almost uniformly fatal, has been much improved by antibiotic treatment, particularly of anaerobic organisms (Weesner and Cisek, 1993). Ligation of the jugular vein has sometimes been performed to prevent thromboembolism.

The following case illustrates an intracranial hypertension caused by thrombosis of the internal jugular vein left lateral sinus and superior sagittal sinus secondary to placement of a long-term intravenous cannula. [This case has also been published by Stephens *et al.* (1991).]

A 48-year-old woman underwent surgical reconstruction of a benign oesophageal stricture. A 14-gauge intravenous cannula was introduced via the brachial vein into the internal jugular vein on each side for infusion of blood and antibiotics: gentamycin, flucloxacillin and metronidazole. On the left side the cannula was left in situ for 5 days for total parenteral nutrition. Nine days after operation a tender inflamed swelling was noted in the region of the mastoid process on the left and the diagnosis of jugular vein thrombosis was confirmed by ultrasound. Anticoagulation was started with heparin followed by warfarin.

Two days later the patient developed headache, vomiting and drowsiness with a low-grade fever and a leucocytosis. Papilloedema and restriction of upward gaze was noted, and a CT scan showed diffuse cerebral swelling and an enhanced scan showed an empty delta sign. It was found that on turning the patient's head to the right she became unresponsive with roving horizontal eye movements. A diagnosis was made of thrombosis of the lateral sinus with propagation to the superior sagittal sinus. Brain swelling was managed successfully with mannitol, acetazolamide and dexamethasone, and warfarin was continued. The neck swelling became indurated and the patient recovered.

This case exhibits a very rare clinical sign more usually associated with occlusive disease of the extracranial arteries – loss of consciousness produced by rotation of the neck. In this case it was probably caused by mechanical compression of the single remaining jugular vein with a subsequent acute rise in intracranial pressure.

4

Causes

INTRODUCTION

The underlying cause of cerebral venous thrombosis still remains undetected in about 20% of cases. The known causes, of which there are now over 100, can be broadly categorized into the three main groups originally proposed by Virchow.

The first group, comprising approximately 70% of the known causes, includes conditions in which there is an increased thrombotic tendency in the blood because of defects, single or combined, of the coagulation mechanism, the fibrinolytic system or in platelet function. These prothrombotic states may be primary inherited disorders or, much more often, secondary to pregnancy, to a haematological or systemic disease, or to the effects of treatment.

In the second, smaller, group, comprising only about 5% of the total, there is a disturbance of blood flow: usually slowing caused by dehydration; increased blood viscosity; mechanical obstruction of veins or sinuses; cardiac failure; or occasionally an excessive blood flow as in an arterio-venous fistula.

The third group comprises a number of diverse conditions causing infection, infiltration or fibrosis of the meninges and walls of the veins or sinuses. It accounts for 12% of known causes. These figures are approximate and are subject to considerable variation according to the age of the patients, the country of origin and the date of the report (Table 4.1).

MECHANISMS OF THROMBOSIS AND PROTHROMBOTIC STATES

The process of thrombosis in veins depends on the interaction of a number of different factors, such as injury to the vessel wall, stagnation of blood flow and hypercoagulability of the blood, which were recognized by Virchow in the last century. Other specific factors such as defects in fibrinolysis have been described more recently. Thrombosis in veins, in contrast to arteries, occurs

Table 4.1 Causes of cerebral venous thrombosis (135 cases) (Bousser 1975–1995)

Cause	Number of cases
Prothrombotic states	**17 (13%)**
Pregnancy	4
Puerperium	13
Inherited thrombophilia	**2 (1.5%)**
Protein S deficiency	1
Antithrombin III deficiency	1
Acquired thrombophilia secondary to blood disorders	**8 (6%)**
Thrombocythaemia	3
Iron deficiency anaemia	2
Primary polycythaemia	1
Paroxysmal nocturnal haemoglobinuria	1
Disseminated intravascular coagulation	1
Thrombophilia secondary to systemic disease	**28 (21%)**
Behçet's disease	18
Breast carcinoma	2
Prostatic carcinoma	1
Lymphoma	1
Systemic lupus erythematosus	2
Nephrotic syndrome	2
Vasculitis	1
Ulcerative colitis	1
Thrombophilia secondary to drugs	**17 (13%)**
Oral contraceptives	14
(Combined with other factors)	15)
Corticosteroids	3
Thrombosis secondary to flow disturbance	**4 (3%)**
Arterio-venous fistula	3
Jugular vein ligation	1
Thrombosis secondary to infection or infiltration	**13 (10%)**
Local	
Otitis	2
Sinusitis	2
Teeth	1
Tonsillitis	1
General	
Carcinomatous meningitis	2
Uveomeningitis	2
Sarcoidosis	1
Chronic meningitis	1
Subdural empyema	1
Miscellaneous causes	**17 (12%)**
Head injury	7
Arachnoid cyst	1
Cholesteatoma	1
Post-operative	1
Von Willebrand's disease	1
Multiple sclerosis	1
Abdominal suppuration	2
Associated venous thrombosis	3
Unknown	**29 (21%)**

under conditions of low flow and venous thrombi are composed of masses of red cells trapped in a fibrin meshwork. Low flow favours formation of thrombosis with a large fibrin component because it allows coagulation factors to reach a high local concentration rather than being rapidly diluted by flowing blood. In the experimental animal, thrombi of this type can be produced by ligation of veins combined with either injury to the vascular endothelium or activation of the coagulation system. Stasis alone is insufficient to induce thrombus formation. In clinical practice the combination of stasis with activation of coagulation and platelet factors, is usually the responsible mechanism.

Thrombosis begins as small aggregates of platelets and fibrin formed on the venous endothelium either at points of minor injury, venostasis or turbulence. In systemic veins regions of stasis are found in association with valves and in the cerebral circulation similar regions of slow or no flow may occur in the lacunae adjacent to the sagittal sinus or in the rugose interstices of the dural sinus walls. The subsequent fate of these aggregates and whether they evolve into larger mixed thrombi, disaggregate or undergo lysis depends on the complex interaction of blood flow, coagulant, anticoagulant and fibrinolytic systems.

PLATELETS

The influence of platelets is much greater in arterial than in venous thrombosis but they are an important initiating factor in both types. Platelets activated either by contact with subendothelial collagen or by thrombin adhere to the venous wall. Adhesion is rapidly followed by aggregation of further platelets under the influence of adenosine diphosphate to form a platelet plug. The early plug is held together by fibrinogen bridges, which rapidly disassociate unless transformed into fibrin by the action of thrombin. Activated platelets accelerate the generation of thrombin by release of Factor V, and by providing phospholipid membrane binding sites for activated Factors X and V. The prothrombinase complex formed on the platelet membrane accelerates the conversion of prothrombin to thrombin.

There are a number of diseases in which an increased thrombotic tendency is caused by abnormal activation of platelets. Some but not all of these may also exhibit thrombocytosis (see Hoch and Silver, 1990, for a review). Myeloproliferative disorders, sepsis, diabetes and hyperlipidaemia all show an increased thrombotic tendency, which is due, at least in part, to this action. Myeloproliferative disorders, which may show both quantitative and qualitative platelet abnormalities, are discussed more fully on page 58.

Abnormal activation of platelets is responsible for the tendency to thrombosis found in patients with hyperlipidaemia, although thrombosis tends to affect arteries rather than veins (Hoch and Silver, 1990). There are a number of possible mechanisms: increased concentration of cholesterol in the platelet membrane of patients with type IIa hyperlipoproteinaemia leads to a heightened sensitivity to aggregating agents. It has been shown *in vitro* that cholesterol loading of platelets results in release of thromboxane and increase in aggregability. Hyperlipidaemia may also activate platelets by changing the reactivity to adenyl cyclase.

The increased thrombotic tendency shown by diabetic patients is also related to changes in platelet activation as well as in vascular endothelium. Release of thromboxane A2, fibrinogen and of von Willebrand's factor from endothelium are all increased in diabetes while platelet sensitivity to prostacycline is decreased. In addition it has been shown that collagen from diabetic patients is a more potent activator of platelets than is collagen from control subjects.

Sepsis increases thrombotic tendency in several ways. Gram-positive bacteria are a direct stimulus to platelet activation. Gram-negative bacteria may have a similar action, but, in addition, they interact with endothelium and leucocytes to express tissue factor and stimulate the coagulation pathway.

COAGULATION MECHANISMS

The 'coagulation cascade' comes into operation when inactive coagulation zymogens are converted into active serine proteases, which then catalyse further zymogen–serine protease conversions. This positive feedback system enables a small stimulus to generate large quantities of thrombin.

The cascade may be initiated by two pathways: an extrinsic pathway triggered by tissue factor in association with Factor VII, and a less important intrinsic pathway triggered by contact activation of Factor XII. The two pathways are not independent, as was once thought, but have complex interactions. The intrinsic pathway is now thought to be more important in regulating fibrinolysis.

The intrinsic pathway begins with the conversion of Factor XII to its active form (XIIa) by interaction with a negatively charged surface such as subendothelial collagen in the presence of high-molecular-weight kallikrein and prekallikrein. Factor XIIa coverts Factor IX to its active form IXa, which in turn activates Factor X in a reaction that takes place on platelet or endothelial cell membranes, and also requires Factor VIIIa and calcium.

The extrinsic pathway is triggered by the release of tissue thromboplastin from injured tissues. Thromboplastin binds to Factor VII in the presence of calcium. The resulting complex is activated by Factors IXa, Xa, and XIIa with a great increase in its proteolytic potential.

In the common pathway, Factor Xa combines with Factor Va and calcium on a phospholipid membrane to form a prothrombinase complex, which catalyses the conversion of prothrombin to thrombin. In a proteolytic reaction, thrombin splits fibrinopeptides A and B from fibrinogen to form fibrin, which then polymerizes into a gel. The final step in the formation of a stable insoluble blood clot is the cross-linking of adjacent fibrin monomers by the action of Factor XIII, activated by thrombin.

NATURAL ANTICOAGULANTS

The coagulation cascade is held in check by three natural anticoagulant proteins: antithrombin III, protein C and heparin cofactor II. Deficiency of natural anticoagulants, which can be inherited or acquired, removes restraints on coagulation and predisposes to thrombosis (see page 54).

Antithrombin III is a serine protease inhibitor that deactivates thrombin, and Factors X and XI, after first forming a complex with a heparin-like substance on the surface of endothelial cells. Protein C is a vitamin K-dependent protein, which is a powerful anticoagulant when converted to its active form, protein Ca. This conversion is brought about by thrombin combining with thrombomodulin on the endothelial surface. Protein Ca cleaves Factors Va and VIIIa, thus preventing formation of the prothrombinase complex. Protein S is a cofactor in this reaction. In addition, protein C enhances fibrinolytic activity (Brookfield, 1974).

A further inherited prothrombotic disorder has been described recently and is much more widespread and more important than simple deficiency of protein C. It is an autosomal dominant mutation in Factor V, which renders Factor V resistant to the effect of activated protein C (Dahlback *et al.*, 1993).

FIBRINOLYSIS

The function of the fibrinolytic system is to remove fibrin and to limit its deposition and fibrinolysis is itself held in check by inhibitors. A prothrombotic state can be produced either by defective fibrinolysis or excessive inhibition.

Activation of the fibrinolytic system causes lysis of fibrin by the action of the enzyme plasmin, which is generated from an inactive precursor plasminogen. Thrombin, as well as converting fibrinogen to fibrin, releases tissue plasminogen activator (tPA) from endothelial cells. tPA and other plasminogen activators convert plasminogen to plasmin on the surface of the thrombus; plasmin then splits fibrin into fibrin degradation products (FDPs). Plasmin formed within a thrombus continues its action for some time but plasmin free in the blood is rapidly inhibited by α_2-plasmin inhibitor.

DISSEMINATED INTRAVASCULAR COAGULATION

Disseminated intravascular coagulation (DIC) is an acquired condition characterized by intravascular coagulation, consumption of platelets and coagulation factors, and secondary activation of the fibrinolytic system. DIC is a complication of a large number of acute disorders including trauma, septicaemia, obstetric infections, liver failure, transfusion reactions and terminal malignant disease. It is often accompanied by cardiorespiratory failure. The common feature to the majority of types of DIC is the abnormal expression of tissue factor on the surfaces of endothelial cells, macrophages and monocytes, leading to activation of the coagulation system by the extrinsic pathway. In some types there is activation of Factor X. Stimulation of fibrinolysis and the fibrinolytic system goes some way to counteract the effects of excessive coagulation, and the outcome of the disease in terms of haemorrhage or ischaemia depends on the balance between these two factors.

A more chronic variety of DIC, seen in patients with cancer, shows that a state of equilibrium can be reached between the activity of the coagulation system and the consumption and replacement of coagulation factors.

CLINICAL PROTHROMBOTIC STATES

CEREBRAL VENOUS THROMBOSIS IN PREGNANCY AND THE PUERPERIUM

Pregnancy or the puerperium is the causative factor most commonly identified in cerebral venous thrombosis and is present in about 20% of patients (Table 4.2). The proportion tends to be higher in underdeveloped countries (Cantu and Barinagarrementeria, 1993). Pregnancy can be considered as a naturally occurring prothrombotic state; in the third trimester and in the puerperium, not only are the levels of procoagulant proteins increased, but fibrinolysis is suppressed by raised levels of plasminogen activator inhibitors and natural anticoagulant substances such as protein S are diminished. The prevalence of thrombosis in any site in association with pregnancy is approximately 1 per 1000 but in the puerperium the figure rises to 4 per 1000 (Carroll *et al.*, 1966).

In physiological conditions, the various factors influencing haemostasis, such as the coagulation system, platelets, vascular endothelium and fibrinolytic system, are in a state of fine balance. There is continuous production of small amounts of procoagulant substances such as activated Factor X and activated Factor V, which combine with platelets to form prothrombinase, which in turn generates thrombin. This process is counteracted by the natural anticoagulants antithrombin III and the protein C/protein S system.

Table 4.2 Thrombosis in pregnancy and puerperium

Prevalence 4 per 1000 (risk increased five-fold), cerebral 1 per 3000

Possible factors: Flow disturbance
- Increased venous distensibility and capacity
- Venous stasis associated with prolonged bed rest, instrumental delivery, haemorrhage, sepsis, multiparity, advanced age

Coagulation/fibrinolytic system disturbance
- Factor II, VII, X increased
- Fibrin generation increased
- Protein S reduced (protein C unchanged)
- Resistance to Protein Ca

Favoured cerebral sites: cortical veins (parieto-occipital), superior sagittal sinus

In individuals with inherited deficiency of these natural anticoagulants, single or repeated episodes of thrombosis usually occur in the second or third decade, sometimes spontaneously, sometimes provoked by pregnancy, oral contraceptives, trauma, surgery or prolonged immobility. Not all patients at risk develop thrombosis; in antithrombin III deficiency the prevalence of thrombosis in pregnancy is about 65% and in protein C deficiency about 25% (Conard *et al.*, 1987).

Although arterial thromboses may also occur, the great majority of patients present with venous events, predominantly in the legs. Protein C or S deficiency is said to affect mainly superficial veins, whereas in antithrombin III deficiency, the deep veins are more often involved.

The strong association of cerebral venous thrombosis with late pregnancy and the puerperium has been noted in some of the earliest descriptions (Collier, 1891). The prevalence of this complication was assessed in 1958 as one in 3000 pregnancies (Huggenberg and Kesselring, 1958) and it accounts for 6% of maternal deaths (Angelov, 1989). In the large series of 73 cases of cerebral venous thrombosis published by Krayenbühl (1967) half occurred during or after pregnancy. Pregnancy-related venous thrombosis occurs at a younger age, has a more abrupt onset, an increased prevalence of anaemia, a decreased mortality (9% vs 33%) and a better chance of full recovery (80% vs 58%) compared to other groups (Cantu and Barinagarrementeria, 1993).

In fatal cases thrombosis is often extensive, involving predominantly the unpaired venous sinuses; rarely the meningeal and intracerebral veins may also be affected. Angelov (1989) has described widespread thrombosis in the cerebral microcirculation, which in some cases was also found in other organs, conforming to the pathological description of DIC. This important observation requires confirmation, since DIC very rarely involves the brain and tends to affect arteries rather than veins. At one time there was thought to be an association with obstetric complications and prolonged labour (Garcin and Pestel, 1949).

Cerebral venous thrombosis in early pregnancy is much less common but has been recorded as early as the eighth week (Lavin and Bone, 1978). The possibility of venous embolism from the pelvic veins to the brain via the vertebral venous plexus was first suggested by Batson (1940) to explain the distribution of metastases and was also favoured by Martin (1944) as a likely factor in the spread of venous thrombi to the brain.

The clinical features of pregnancy-related cerebral venous thrombosis conform to the classical description given above (King, 1950). The onset is most frequently from 1–20 days after delivery and a smaller number of patients in the second or third trimester (Eon *et al.*, 1989). Conard *et al.* (1990) reported an overall prevalence of venous thrombosis in antithrombin III-deficient women of 44% with no significant difference in risk between pregnancy and the puerperium. In protein C and S deficiency, however, the number of cases during pregnancy is small and the risk is significantly greater in the puerperium. There is no association with toxaemia of pregnancy or with hypertension.

The favoured site for pregnancy-related cerebral venous thrombosis appears to be the superior sagittal sinus and related cortical veins, particularly in the parieto-occipital region (Martin, 1944). Thrombosis may spread to the major anastomotic cortical veins of Labbé and Trolard thereby increasing the risk of cerebral infarction and haemorrhage. Internal cerebral veins including the great vein of Galen may also be involved (Barre and Grenier, 1932; Krenz and Power, 1990). The early symptoms are headache, vomiting and loss of alertness followed by focal or generalized seizures, and by focal signs of hemiparesis, hemisensory disturbance or hemianopia. Marked fluctuation in the physical signs from minute to minute is characteristic; alternating hemiparesis changing from one side to the other over hours is rare but strongly suggests a venous thrombosis (Barre and Grenier, 1932). The level of consciousness is also variable; the spinal fluid is clear or bloodstained, and is under increased pressure.

INHERITED PROTHROMBOTIC DISORDERS (Table 4.3)

Protein C and S deficiency

Protein C is a naturally occurring serine protease with a similar structure to Factors VII, IX and X. It acts as an anticoagulant by virtue of its ability to inactivate Factors V and VIII. When thrombin binds on to the endothelial surface receptor, thrombomodulin, the resulting complex, activates protein C, which acts as a negative feedback mechanism and limits the spread of intravascular thrombosis. Protein S is a cofactor for the activation of protein C and deficiency of either protein is associated with a tendency to thrombosis, usually venous. Approximately 20% of patients having venous thrombo-embolism below age 45 have been shown to be deficient in protein C, S or antithrombin III; a further 1–2% show abnormalities of thrombin production caused by plasminogen deficiency or by abnormal varieties of fibrin resistant to dissolution by plasmin (Brookfield, 1974).

There is a poor correlation between levels of these factors and the occurrence of thrombosis. In the patient described by Cros *et al.* (1990), protein S was undetectable in the patient, who had suffered from multiple thrombotic events since adolescence, and in his father, who was symptomless.

The underlying cause of thrombophilia in the remaining 80% of patients was unknown until the recent discovery of a second factor involving protein C (Dahlbäck *et al.*, 1993). This defect is also familial, inherited as an autosomal dominant trait and produces a prothrombotic state in which there is resistance to activated protein C, correctable by normal plasma. The defect is a mutation in factor V (Factor V Leiden). This appears to account for about half the previously unknown cases and may prove to be the most important cause of familial thrombophilia (Koster *et al.*, 1993; Kimberet *et al.*, 1996). Five of 25 patients with cerebral venous thrombosis cited by Martinelli *et al.* (1996) showed this abnormality compared with 2.7% of controls (see also pages 134–5).

The homozygous form of protein C deficiency causes extensive dermal

Table 4.3 Inherited prothrombotic disorders

Disease	Suggested mechanism
Protein C deficiency	↓ natural anticoagulant inhibiting Factor V
Protein S deficiency	↓ cofactor for protein C
Factor Va resistance (Leiden mutation)	Factor Va resistant to action of protein C
Antithrombin III deficiency	↓ inactivation of thrombin
Familial plasminogen defect	↓ fibrinolysis
Homocystinuria	Vascular endothelial injury ↑ platelet deposition

↓, decreased; ↑, increased.

haemorrhage in the neonatal period and is usually incompatible with survival. Most patients in clinical practice have heterozygous familial deficiency of protein C or S. An acquired form of the deficiency may occur in liver disease, disseminated intravascular coagulation and during warfarin therapy. A transient relative deficiency also may occur following surgery. In the case of the Leiden mutation, homozygous individuals may be unaffected, suggesting incomplete penetrance (for review, see Hajjar, 1994).

Cases of cerebral venous thrombosis associated with protein C or S deficiency have been reported in young adults or children, usually female, often with a history of venous thrombosis in the legs and sometimes on oral contraceptive drugs. Deficiency of protein C has been cited as a cause of cerebral venous thrombosis more frequently than protein S. The superior sagittal sinus appears to be the site most often affected. The presentation can be as benign intracranial hypertension (Enevoldson and Ross Russell, 1990) or cortical venous infarction (Vieregge *et al.*, 1989). Additional provoking factors, such as pregnancy, oral contraceptive drugs or head trauma are often present (Heistinger *et al.*, 1992; Rich *et al.*, 1993). An unusually severely affected patient reported by Wintzen *et al.* (1985) had haemorrhagic infarction of the choroid plexus causing obstructive hydrocephalus. In some cases, deficiency of protein S may be combined with other prothrombotic factors such as a raised fibrinogen concentration (Pasquale *et al.*, 1990).

Antithrombin III deficiency

Substances synthesized by vascular endothelium also have a powerful influence on the coagulation mechanism. Antithrombin III (ATIII), potentiated by the action of heparin (also synthesized by endothelium), binds irreversibly to the active site of thrombin and every other serine protease coagulation factor, thus inactivating them. This process can occur either at sites of injury to the vessel wall or during spontaneous thrombosis within the lumen. ATIII deficiency is thought to account for about 2% of adult venous thrombosis. A thrombotic tendency occurs when levels of antithrombin III are reduced below 60% of normal. There appears to be either a quantitative deficiency of ATIII or an abnormal molecule. The disorder is inherited as an autosomal dominant trait. In an affected individual, the thrombotic tendency usually affects the venous system in the legs and appears in early adult life often following infections, trauma, burns or childbirth. Pulmonary embolism and arterial thromboses have been reported but are rare; the risk of thrombosis in pregnancy is about 70%.

Cerebral venous thrombosis affecting the superficial venous system of the cerebral hemisphere and resulting in a haemorrhagic infarction of the temporal lobe was reported in a 15-year-old boy with a strong family history of venous thrombosis (Ambruso *et al.*, 1980). Treatment with long-term anticoagulation using warfarin was successful. A similar instance was reported by Sauron *et al.* (1982) in which the patient suffered a cerebellar event, an unusual site for venous infarction.

Concentrates of protein C and antithrombin III are now available for the treatment of patients with inherited deficiencies, and are used at times of high risk of thrombosis, such as in pregnancy or after surgery, with or without additional heparin. In the presence of low levels of antithrombin III, heparin alone is relatively ineffective. Warfarin is suitable for long-term prophylaxis.

Inherited disorders of fibrinolysis

Quantitative or qualitative defects in plasminogen activity have been held responsible for some varieties of familial thrombophilia. Isaacson and Nilsson (1972) found impaired fibrinolysis in blood and vein walls in no less than 70% of patients with deep venous thrombosis in the legs. In about half the cases there was reduced plasminogen activity with normal concentration of the antigen; in half there was reduced plasminogen concentration. There is little indication that abnormalities in fibrinolysis account for many cases of cerebral venous thrombosis. A single well-documented case was reported by Schutta *et al.* (1991). The patient was a man of 34 who presented with symptoms of raised intracranial pressure and cerebral oedema and was found to have widespread thrombosis of intracranial veins, including both internal jugular veins and the sagittal sinus. Plasminogen activity was 58% of that found in pooled plasma (normal 75–130%) and plasminogen antigen concentration measured by electroimmunoassay was 50%. Subnormal levels were also found in his father and daughter. Other possible prothrombotic factors were thrombocytosis and hyperthyroidism. The patient recovered and recanalization of the sagittal sinus was demonstrated some months later.

Homocystinuria

Of the various conditions causing homocystinuria, much the most important is an inherited deficiency of cystathionine B synthase, an enzyme essential for the formation of normal cross-linkages in collagen. It is inherited as an autosomal recessive trait. Homozygotes have high levels of homocysteine and methionine in the plasma, and homocystine in the urine. The diagnosis is made by a positive nitroprusside reaction in the urine or by showing the enzyme deficiency in cultured skin fibroblasts.

Affected patients have a Marfanoid habitus, ectopia lentis, osteoporosis, fair hair, skeletal deformity and mild mental retardation. There is also a strong tendency to premature cardiovascular disease and to thromboses, both arterial and venous (Heijer *et al.*, 1995). This is thought to be caused by homocystine-induced injury to vascular endothelium, which progresses to platelet deposition and thrombosis. Abnormal platelet adhesiveness may be a further factor.

Although the majority of reported cases have had arterial occlusions, there are a significant number with venous thromboses, including the dural sinuses. The first patient to be recognized with the disease had a sagittal sinus thrombosis, and more recent cases have been reported in young patients presenting with raised intracranial pressure by Cochran and Packman (1992) and by Mohamed *et al.* (1991). Treatment is by dietary restriction of methionine and in some cases the metabolic abnormality can be partially reversed by pyridoxin. The diagnosis of homocystinuria should be considered in patients who present with cerebral sinus or venous disease in early life.

ACQUIRED PROTHROMBOTIC STATES SECONDARY TO BLOOD DISORDERS

A tendency to thrombosis may be a feature of various acquired blood disorders. The underlying causes are often obscure and multiple; in some there may be quantitative or qualitative platelet defects, in others there may be abnormal activation of the coagulation system. Physical factors such as stasis or increased blood viscosity may also play an important part.

MYELOPROLIFERATIVE DISEASES

These comprise a group of clonal stem-cell disorders of the bone marrow and include primary proliferative polycythaemia (polycythaemia rubra vera), primary (essential) thrombocythaemia, chronic myeloid leukaemia and chronic myelofibrosis. In these disorders there are increased numbers of red cells, white cells and platelets, but, in addition, the megekaryocytes in the bone marrow are defective, resulting in the production of platelets that are qualitatively abnormal. These defects include deranged ultrastructure, loss of adrenergic, prostaglandin and Fc receptors, abnormal arachidonic acid metabolism, and acquired storage pool disease.

Patients with myeloproliferative disorders show an increased tendency to both venous and arterial thromboses, including those occurring in unusual sites such as splenic, portal, mesenteric and hepatic veins, and in the cerebral veins and sinuses.

Table 4.4 Prothrombotic blood disorders

Disease	Suggested mechanism
Polycythaemia vera	↑ blood viscosity, slowed flow ↑ platelets Abnormal platelet behaviour
Primary thrombocythaemia	↑ platelets Abnormal platelet behaviour
Leukaemias	↑ viscosity Meningeal infiltration Effects of treatment (asparginase)
Sickle cell disease	↑ viscosity Venous endothelial damage
Haemolytic anaemias, paroxysmal nocturnal haemoglobinuria	Haemolysis ↑ thromboplastin release

↑, increased.

Polycythaemia

Polycythaemia denotes an increased red cell count, haemoglobin level or packed cell volume, and can be divided into two main groups, absolute and apparent. True polycythaemia consists of polycythaemia rubra vera, a myeloproliferative disorder of unknown cause and the secondary polycythaemias, which result from a variety of different stimuli, such as hypoxaemia and renal disease. In absolute polycythaemia, the red cell mass is increased, whereas in apparent polycythaemia the red cell count and packed cell volume are raised because of a reduction in plasma volume, the red cell mass remaining normal. The abnormal thrombotic tendency found in many types of polycythaemia is partly the result of the slowing of blood flow from increased viscosity and partly due to changes in platelet numbers or function. Polycythaemia rubra vera is caused by excessive proliferation of a pluripotent progenitor cell, which has the potential to develop into red cell granulocytes or platelets. Erythropoietin levels are normal or reduced, but red cell precursors *in vitro* have an exaggerated dose response to erythropoietin. Myelofibrotic transformation is usually the end-stage of the disease in those patients who survive long enough. Acute leukaemia occurs in up to 13% of patients.

The packed cell volume (PCV) is the major determinant of whole blood viscosity, which increases markedly at levels of PCV over 0.52; white cells and other plasma constituents such as fibrinogen also have a significant but much smaller effect. If blood flow through an organ such as the brain is measured at different levels of PCV, it decreases in a linear fashion as the PCV rises. Oxygen transport, calculated by the product of blood flow and oxygen content, is optimum at levels of haematocrit between 0.40 and 0.50. Above this level adequate levels of oxygen transport can only be achieved by compensatory mechanisms such as an increased plasma volume or cardiac output, or a decreased peripheral resistance. In patients with cerebral or coronary artery disease these mechanisms may be inadequate. In addition to the effects of increased blood viscosity, the increased number and abnormal behaviour of platelets, which often accompanies polycythaemia rubra vera, are additional prothrombotic factors leading to occlusion of both large and small cerebral blood vessels and to spontaneous platelet aggregation *in vivo*. Finally there is defective haemostasis, also due to abnormal platelet morphology or membrane function, which may lead to the paradox of both thrombotic and haemorrhagic tendencies in the same patient.

In polycythaemia rubra vera, cerebral vascular occlusions are five times commoner than in the general population and the risk of such events has been shown to be proportional to the rise in PCV (Schafer, 1984). Of 511 patients reviewed by Silverstein *et al.* (1962), 48 had cerebral vascular lesions, either ischaemic or haemorrhagic, and these were the presenting symptoms in 17. Many of the haemorrhagic infarcts were probably caused by cortical vein or sinus occlusion, although this was not proven. Three patients had raised intracranial pressure suggesting sagittal sinus obstruction. Similar reports of haemorrhagic infarction and raised intracranial pressure from thrombosis of the sagittal and cavernous sinuses in patients with mixed myeloproliferative disorders have appeared recently (Haan *et al.*, 1988). Some of these patients had increased platelet count and megakaryopoesis as part of polycythaemia rubra vera. There appeared to be little correlation between quantitative or qualitative platelet abnormality and the risk of thrombosis. Two instances of cavernous sinus thrombosis following thrombosis of the intracranial internal carotid artery have been reported in patients with polycythaemia rubra vera (Melamed *et al.*, 1976). The suggested mechanism was occlusion of small branches of the internal carotid supplying the walls of the cavernous sinus. Heparin-induced thrombocytopenia was held responsible for cerebral venous thrombosis in a patient with polycythaemia reported by Kyritsis *et al.* (1990).

Secondary hypoxaemic polycythaemia may be a factor in the susceptibility of children with congenital heart disease to cerebral sino-venous thrombosis, as the majority of reported cases are in those with cyanotic disease. Polycythaemia as a result of altitude may also be a cause of cerebral venous thrombosis. Fujimaki *et al.* (1986) reported the case of a young man presenting with signs of raised intracranial presure and brain oedema. Haemoglobin concentration was 21.5 g dl^{-1}. Haemorrhagic cerebral infarction was found at surgery with thrombosis of cortical veins.

Primary Thrombocythaemia

This is a variety of myeloproliferative disorder in which there is hyperplasia of megakaryocytes and an increase in the platelet count. There may also be some increase in granulocytes. Characteristically the platelet count is greater than 600×10^9 l^{-1} but counts as high as 2500×10^9 l^{-1} may be found. In reactive thrombocytosis it is unusual for counts to rise above 1000×10^9 l^{-1}. In primary thrombocythaemia the platelets are morphologically abnormal with many large and bizarre forms. There is an increased thrombotic tendency but, in addition, haemorrhage may occur because of functional platelet defects shown *in vitro* by decreased aggregation on exposure to agents such as adrenalin or ADP. Conversely there may be spontaneous platelet aggregation *in vivo*, visible in the retinal microcirculation, and a defective response to the inhibitory prostaglandin PGI2. The usual clinical features are episodes of ischaemia or haemorrhage, ischaemia being much the commoner. Thrombosis may involve femoral or splenic veins with embolism to the lungs. Thrombosis of digital arteries causing small areas of gangrene on the tips of the fingers is a characteristic feature. Bleeding may occur in the skin, the alimentary tract or (rarely) the renal tract.

Haan *et al.*, 1988 have described two patients with cerebral venous thrombosis as a presenting feature of idiopathic thrombocythaemia. Both had haemorrhagic cerebral infarction caused by thrombosis of cortical veins, and one had, in addition, intracranial hypertension and sagittal sinus thrombosis. The authors found a poor correlation between platelet numbers and thrombosis, and also questioned the value of qualitative tests of platelet function. As with other prothrombotic disorders, the onset of thrombosis may be provoked by other influences such as pregnancy (R. Ross Russell, unpublished observation).

The course of the disease is variable but is frequently benign, especially in young patients or in those in whom the platelet abnormality is discovered by chance. Agents such as hydroxyurea, interferon and low-dose alkylating agents have been used to control the disease, which has a median survival of 10–12 years.

LEUKAEMIA

In acute leukaemia the large increase in white cells may produce an increase in viscosity with stasis and impaction of masses of cells in the microcirculation producing microinfarcts. There is also a tendency to massive haemorrhage during blastic crises with white cell counts in excess of 300 000 mm^{-3}. In the brain leukaemic deposits may be found within vessels or infiltrating meninges, nerve roots and parenchyma.

There have been a number of reports of dural sinus thrombosis in children with acute lymphoblastic leukaemia. David *et al.* (1975) described a 7-year-old boy who died following raised intracranial hypertension. The brain was found to be normal but the sagittal sinus was occluded with thrombus, and the walls of the sinus infiltrated with blast cells. Steinherz *et al.* (1981) in a review and report of two further cases estimated cerebral venous thrombosis to have a prevalence of 1% in acute lymphoblastic leukaemia, possibly related to asparginase-induced antithrombin III deficiency. Chronic raised intracranial pressure without cerebral infarction appears to be the usual mode of presentation.

SICKLE CELL DISEASE

Individuals who inherit the gene for haemoglobin S may be homozygous or heterozygous. In the homozygous form, 90% of haemoglobin is HbS and the patient suffers from sickle cell anaemia. In the heterozygous form, HbS comprises 50% of the total, the remainder being HbA. Red cells containing HbS are more rigid than normal and have a shortened life span. The main factors that underlie the degree of red-cell flexibility are the proportion of HbS and the oxygen tension. The precipitation of insoluble HbS within the red cell at reduced oxygen tensions leads to 'sickling' of the red cells and loss of the normal flexibility.

About 10% of individuals with sickle cell (SS) anaemia suffer some type of neurological event, usually in childhood and, as a rule, consisting of cerebral infarction following occlusion or stenoses of large arteries. Subarachnoid or intracranial haemorrhage may also occur. Subendothelial fibroblast proliferation in arteries of the circle of Willis may lead to extensive development of collateral vessels (moya-moya disease). Venous thrombosis is unusual but has been recorded (Vernant *et al.*, 1988; Garcia, 1990). It is suggested that damage to the walls of arteries and veins results from sickle-cell 'sludging' in the small vessels of the vasa vasorum. Extensive thrombosis of the deep venous system causing bilateral thalamic infarction in a 2-year-old child with sickle cell anaemia is recorded (Oguz *et al.*, 1994).

Patients with sickle cell trait usually suffer no clinical disability but may develop complications when exposed to severely hypoxic conditions. As in sickle cell disease, clumps of sickled red cells may block small blood vessels and, in addition, there may be thrombosis of small and medium-sized arteries and veins. Schenk (1964) reported one of the first cases of sinus thrombosis in a 12-year-old boy with sickle cell trait who developed seizures, hemiparesis and raised intracranial pressure shortly after tonsillectomy. Death occurred after a month and at autopsy there was extensive brain oedema and thrombosis of the sagittal sinus.

PAROXYSMAL NOCTURNAL HAEMOGLOBINURIA

Paroxysmal nocturnal haemoglobinuria (PNH) is a rare non-familial disorder causing a chronic haemolytic anaemia beginning in the third or fourth decade. It is an acquired genetic disorder, owing to a mutation in a primitive precursor blood cell in bone marrow. Affected red cells are abnormally sensitive to the lytic action of complement and platelets are more sensitive than normal to complement-mediated platelet activation. The defective gene, PIG-A, is situated on the X chromosome (Miyata *et al.*, 1994). Haemolysis occurs particularly during sleep accompanied by chest or abdominal pain and haemoglobinuria. The commonest cause of death is cerebral or abdominal venous thrombosis or pulmonary embolism. There is a macrocytic anaemia with a high reticulocyte count and leucopenia; bone marrow failure may occur.

The diagnosis is made by the acidified serum (Ham) test. Affected patients have a strong tendency to develop venous thrombosis, thought to be caused by release of thromboplastic material from haemolysed erythrocytes.

In a recent series of 80 patients, mean age at diagnosis was 42 years and median survival was 10 years; 28% were still alive after 25 years, 10% having made a spontaneous recovery (Hillman *et al.*, 1995). In the same report, there were four instances of cerebral venous thrombosis compared with 17 of intra-abdominal thromboses and nine of pulmonary embolism. Arterial stroke occurred in two patients.

Long-term anticoagulant treatment is used to prevent venous thromboses; platelet transfusions may be necessary if there is thrombocytopenia and haemorrhage, and aplasia may require bone-marrow transplantation.

Johnson *et al.* (1970) reported a fatal case of PNH affecting a 49-year-old man presenting with headache, vomiting and hemisensory disturbance. Symptoms began in one leg and progressed to a severe hemiplegia caused by thrombosis of a cortical vein. Death occurred from widespread thrombosis including the inferior vena cava. Patients with cerebral venous thrombosis but without focal neurological signs have also been cited (Al-Hakim *et al.*, 1993).

OTHER TYPES OF ANAEMIA

There are scattered reports of non-infectious sinus or venous thrombosis in other varieties of anaemia. Sagittal sinus thrombosis may occur after acute surgical blood loss or, more commonly, after chronic uterine or rectal bleeding and severe iron deficiency. There may or may not be a thrombocytosis (Stehle *et al.*, 1991). The first recorded case of fatal internal cerebral vein thrombosis was in a 20-year-old girl with chlorosis (iron deficiency anaemia) (Andrew, 1865); Johnsen *et al.* (1973) documented internal cerebral vein thrombosis in a 16-month-old infant with iron deficiency anaemia and further examples involving superficial veins and sinuses were reported by Dickinson (1896). Kalbag and Woolf (1967) reviewed a number of similar cases from the early European literature; it is striking that these were exclusively in young women and comprised about one third of the total number of cases of cerebral venous thrombosis reported at that time. Multiple sinus thromboses, including both the superficial and deep venous systems, have also resulted from severe nutritional iron deficiency in infants (Belman *et al.*, 1990). Haemolytic anaemia was mentioned as a possible cause of sino-venous thrombosis in the large series of cases collected by Krayenbühl (1967) and by Sjolin (1959) in a child with osteopetrosis. In this case, however, osteomyelitis of the facial bones was present and thrombosis may have been infective.

CRYOFIBRINOGENAEMIA

Cryofibrinogen is a variety of fibrinogen, which is soluble at 37°C but precipitates as a gel at 4°C. Increased amounts of cryofibrinogen may be found in patients with neoplasms, notably of the kidney or ovary, in myeloproliferative disorders, in ulcerative colitis and in hypothyroidism. The condition may also be idiopathic. The clinical effects are diverse and include neuropathy, Raynaud's syndrome, gastrointestinal bleeding, and leg vein thrombosis, particularly on exposure to cold. Dunsker *et al.* (1970) reported a patient with a fibrinogen concentration of 6 g l^{-1} of which 1 g was cryofibrinogen. He had a history of leg vein thrombosis on exposure to cold and later developed symptoms of intracranial hypertension with headache, papilloedema and a cerebrospinal fluid (CSF) pressure of 33 cm. Angiography showed thrombosis of the sigmoid sinus and extensive collateral channels. The illness ran a 2-year fatal course with death from thrombosis of the inferior vena cava and renal veins.

PROTHROMBOTIC STATES ACCOMPANYING SYSTEMIC DISEASE OR TREATMENT

Venous thrombosis may be an important feature of a number of diverse systemic diseases (Table 4.5) and in some it may be the presenting symptom. Although the veins of the legs or pelvis are most often affected the cerebral veins and sinuses may also be involved. Thrombosis may also follow the use of drugs or hormone treatment (Table 4.6). Although in some of these conditions the abnormal factors leading to thrombosis have been identified, in many the cause remains obscure.

THROMBOSIS AS A NON-METASTATIC COMPLICATION OF MALIGNANT DISEASE

It has been known since the time of Trousseau that systemic venous thrombosis, especially affecting the pelvic or leg veins, is a frequent complication of malignant disease with a prevalence of 5–15% in all neoplasms and up to 50% in pancreatic or mucin-secreting carcinomas. Although a number of haematological abnormalities have been described, the cause is still uncertain, and there is often the added possibility that chemotherapy, hormones or steroids may be partly responsible. Possible causative factors are an increased synthesis of thromboplastin-like substances by monocytes and macrophages, stimulated by tumour antigens; this has been shown in patients with myeloma and mucin-secreting adenocarcinoma. Proteases may be produced by tumours of breast, colon or vagina, which may activate Factor X in the coagulation system directly; neoplastic cells may also increase platelet activation.

Other abnormal findings in cancer patients include elevated levels of fibrinogen, Factors V, VIII, IX and XI, decreased concentration of antithrombin III, and increased turnover of fibrinogen and platelets. Conversely fibrinolysis may also be increased leading to an increased tendency to haemorrhage. In cancer patients, it appears that there is activation of both coagulation and

Table 4.5 Prothrombotic states secondary to systemic disease

Disease	Suggested mechanism
Malignant disease	↑ thromboplastin (secreted by monocytes, macrophages) Tumour proteases – Factor Xa ↑ fibrinogen ↑ Factors V, VIII, IX, XI ↓ Antithrombin (AT III) Effects of treatment
Inflammatory bowel disease	↑ thromboplastin ↑ platelets ↑ Factors III, V, VIII ↓ ATIII Effects of treatment
Nephrotic syndrome	↑ platelets ↑ Factors V, VIII ↓ ATIII, protein C, plasminogen
Systemic lupus erythematosus	↑ lupus anticoagulant, aPL ↓ protein C, S, ATIII ↓ fibrinolysis ↑ fibrinogen Platelets abnormal

↑, increased; ↓, decreased.

Table 4.6 Drug-induced cerebral venous thrombosis

Drug	Suggested mechanism
Oral contraceptives	↑ fibrinogen ↑ Factors II, VII, VIII, IX, X ↓ antithrombin III (AT III), ↓ fibrinolysis
Corticosteroids	↑ Factors VIII, IX
ε-Aminocaproic acid	↓ plasmin activity
L-Asparginase	↓ plasma proteins, including protein C, protein S and ATIII

↑, increased; ↓, decreased.

fibrinolytic systems combined with decreased anticoagulant activity, and the clinical expression depends on the balance between these factors.

Diagnostic confusion may arise when dural sinuses or cortical veins become thrombosed in the presence of malignant disease, but in the absence of local pathology (paraneoplastic syndrome). This was first pointed out by Averback (1978) and later reviewed by Hickey *et al.* (1982). These patients may present with seizures or haemorrhagic cerebral infarction and show venous thrombosis, often in multiple sites in the brain and elsewhere. In one of the patients described by Averback and in the patient with carcinoma of the gall bladder described by Smith *et al.* (1983) anaplastic tumour cells were detected infiltrating vascular walls and within the organizing thrombus in the superior sagittal sinus and the cortical veins. Both superficial and deep cerebral venous systems may be involved. Cancer of the lung or breast, or acute lymphoblastic leukaemia were again the commonest underlying lesions.

ULCERATIVE COLITIS

Venous thrombosis is a significant complication of severe ulcerative colitis. Clinically evident thrombosis occurs in 1.2–7.5% of cases but evidence of thrombosis at autopsy is much higher – 32–39%. The sites of thrombosis include veins of the pelvis, lungs, spleen and kidneys, and an acute thrombophlebitis of the thoracoepigastric vein is characteristic. The thrombotic tendency has been variously ascribed to accelerated thromboplastin generation, thrombocytosis, increased Factors III, V and VIII, increased fibrinogen, decreased antithrombin III, decreased Protein S, or to the effects of corticosteroid treatment (Yerby and Bailey, 1980; Vaezi *et al.*, 1995). Although cerebral venous thrombosis is rare, increasing numbers of cases are being reported, since it was first observed by Harrison and Truelove (1987) in 2 out of 800 patients with the disease in Oxford (Das *et al.*, 1996; Silburn *et al.*, 1996). There may be a fatal outcome; a patient with fulminating ulcerative colitis and thrombocytosis with multiple thrombosis in lungs, kidneys and prostatic plexus developed headache, stupor and hemiparesis, and died from severe brain swelling, which was unresponsive to mannitol or steroids. At autopsy there was generalized brain oedema with thrombosis of all the venous sinuses and surface veins, and a haemorrhagic infarct in the parieto-occipital region. Microscopic examination showed that even the small intracerebral venules were thrombosed (Borda *et al.*, 1973). Excision of the diseased segment of bowel does not remove the risk of thrombosis and a patient has been recorded with sagittal sinus thrombosis 10 years after proctocolectomy (Yerby and Bailey, 1980).

Other forms of inflammatory bowel disease notably regional enteritis (Crohn's disease) have also been followed by cerebral venous thrombosis (Motte *et al.*, 1992).

NEPHROTIC SYNDROME

A thrombotic tendency to both arterial and venous thrombosis is a recognized feature of the children with the nephrotic syndrome. Various explanations have been put forward including thrombocytosis and elevated levels of Factors V and VIII. The loss of natural anticoagulant or thrombolytic proteins such as Protein S, antithrombin III or plasminogen in the urine as a result of heavy proteinuria is also likely to be a significant factor (Laversuch *et al.*, 1995), and the urinary concentration of these proteins has been shown to be raised. Disseminated intravascular coagulation with decreased levels of fibrinogen and fibrin degradation products may also occur.

Many of the larger series of patients with cerebral venous thrombosis contain cases secondary to nephrotic syndromes (Bousser *et al.*, 1985). Lau *et al.* (1980) reported a 2-year-old child with nephrotic syndrome who developed thrombosis of the sagittal sinus, cortical veins and femoral artery. The presenting clinical features were drowsiness and irritability, followed by a left-sided seizure and hemiparesis. A good recovery followed heparin treatment.

An affected child who died after massive pulmonary embolism from sagittal sinus thrombosis was shown to have a marked deficiency of Factor XII (Delmas *et al.*, 1992). In another case, a 3-year-old child with intracranial hypertension and nephrotic syndrome, there was complete remission after treatment with low-dose heparin and fresh-frozen plasma (Freycon *et al.*, 1992).

SYSTEMIC LUPUS ERYTHEMATOSUS

Systemic lupus erythematosus (SLE) is a multisystem disease in which tissue damage is caused by circulating autoantibodies. It has a prevalence rate of 1 per 2000 in the USA and is commoner in blacks than whites. The cause is unknown but some types may be drug induced. The presence of increased amounts of gammaglobulin and elevated titres of viral antibody as well as non-organ-specific autoantibodies are indications of B-lymphocyte overactivity. The formation of antigen–antibody complexes activates the complement cascade, which itself causes increased vascular permeability and promotes an inflammatory response. Circulating immune complexes are detectable in the serum and deposition of complexes can be detected by immunofluoresence or electron microscopy.

The clinical features are diverse and relapsing, and the systems involved, in order of frequency, are musculo-articular, cutaneous, neurological, renal, pulmonary and cardiac. General complaints, such as fever, fatigue and weight loss are frequent. The commonest neurological symptoms are headache, seizures and a fluctuating organic confusional state, sometimes with psychotic features. Some patients have abrupt focal stroke-like disturbances of cerebral function, with localized lesions resembling infarction on brain scanning. Histological examination may show occlusion of small arteries with platelet or hyaline thrombi, but there is seldom any evidence of true vasculitis within the vessel wall.

The occurrence of vascular cerebral lesions is strongly correlated with the presence of lupus anticoagulant, a group of acquired circulating gamma-immunoglobulins, IgG, IgM or mixed. There are complex interactions between lupus anticoagulant and endothelial cells that may lead to depletion of protein C and S, and a prothrombotic state. Other possible factors are defective fibrinolysis, depletion of antithrombin III and increased fibrinogenaemia.

Vidailhet *et al.* (1990) have given the best account of cerebral venous thrombosis occurring in SLE. They found six examples from a total of 400 patients. The great majority were young women who had suffered from SLE for about 15 years. In only one patient was venous thrombosis the presenting feature. Most of the patients had neurological symptoms other than those caused by venous disease. Five of the six patients had an acute stroke-like onset with a focal deficit in four. Three had seizures and one the features of benign intracranial hypertension. Headache was a symptom in all patients. The sagittal sinus was occluded in five cases and the cortical veins in one.

The prognosis for patients with SLE has greatly improved since immunosuppressive therapy with steroids and cyclophosphamide has been combined with anticoagulants. This also applies to those with venous thrombosis and post-thrombotic recanalization of the sagittal sinus has been demonstrated. The outlook is not always favourable, however. Leslie *et al.* (1987) published an account of a patient who developed widespread sinus thrombosis 9 months after the first symptoms of SLE. She died of cerebral oedema with haemorrhagic infarcts in both hemispheres and cerebellum. A unique feature of this case was the finding of marked vasculitis of the meningeal veins with a polymorph cellular reaction and necrosis of the walls. The arteries showed no vasculitis.

ANTIPHOSPHOLIPID ANTIBODY SYNDROME

Antiphospholipid antibodies (aPL) are a diverse group of acquired circulating immunoglobulins of varied IgG and IgM composition. They include lupus anticoagulant (LA) and anticardiolipin antibody. These were first described in association with SLE, but were shown more recently to occur in patients without features of autoimmune disease but with a multisystem prothrombotic state affecting arteries and veins of all sizes (Hughes, 1993). They occur mainly but not exclusively in young patients with a female : male ratio of 2 : 1. Recurrent spontaneous abortion is another common feature. Neurological episodes include stroke-like attacks, multiple-infarct dementia, migraine, chorea, epilepsy and transverse myelopathy. Livedo reticularis, hypertension, and ischaemic and valvular heart disease have often been recorded. Veins of the leg are most frequently involved, but thrombosis may also affect retinal, pulmonary, renal and hepatic veins. There is sometimes thrombocytopenia and a false-positive serological reaction for syphilis. In addition, many patients show raised levels of antinuclear antibody, LA, IgG and IgM anticardiolipin antibodies.

It has been claimed that 7% of all patients with stroke are aPL positive (Montalban *et al.*, 1991), but some of these reports lack a control group and there are no prospective or cohort studies. This is important because the prevalence of positive antiphospholipid antibodies in the general population is still uncertain (Muir, 1995). A further source of confusion is the reporting of aPL as either positive or negative, positive being greater than two standard deviations above the mean and including by definition 2.5% of the control population.

Anticardiolipin, usually in low titre, is found in up to 7.5% of the normal population, especially in the elderly and in association with autoimmune diseases, and bacterial and viral infections, including AIDS and malignant tumours. The titre of aPL is not clearly related to the risk of thrombosis and immunosuppressive therapy does not appear to reduce the incidence of vascular events (see Muir, 1995, for review).

The mechanism of thrombosis is still speculative. It is suggested that vascular endothelial damage leads to the exposure of anionic phospholipid surfaces. β2 glycoprotein binds to phospholipid which then becomes immunogenic and stimulates the formation of antiphospholipid antibodies.

Cerebral venous thrombosis in association with LA was described by Levine *et al.* (1987) in two patients, including a young pregnant woman with a history of spontaneous abortion, femoral thrombosis and pulmonary embolism who developed raised intracranial pressure following a transverse sinus thrombosis. The second patient had ataxia, diplopia and headache with partial thrombosis of sagittal and transverse sinuses. A further example of a patient presenting with persistent headache and thrombocytopenia was cited by Agah *et al.*, (1996). There are few reports of vascular pathology in the antiphospholipid syndrome; thrombosis of cerebral vessels has been described but there is no evidence of vasculitis (Levine *et al.*, 1987).

Although an immunologically mediated prothrombotic state appears to be a feature of both SLE and the antiphospholipid syndrome, it is still not clear why occlusion of large and medium-sized cerebral arteries occurs more frequently in the antiphospholipid syndrome and why thrombosis in the veins is relatively uncommon.

In Sjögren's syndrome (keratoconjunctivitis sicca), neurological complications have a prevalence of about 20% mainly in the form of spinal cord lesions and polyradiculopathy. There may be a lymphocytic meningitis, which may involve the meningeal vessels and sometimes a necrotizing arteritis. Small veins in cerebral white matter may show inflammatory changes but thrombosis is unusual unless the patient also has antiphospholipid antibodies (Urban *et al.*, 1994)

THROMBOPHLEBITIS MIGRANS AND BUERGER'S DISEASE

Many of the early reports on spontaneous recurrent thrombophlebitis involving femoral, pelvic and visceral veins were probably examples of familial thrombophilia caused by one of the coagulation defects described above (Moorhead and Abramson, 1928). Some of these reports describe cerebral venous thrombosis, usually occurring after many episodes of femoral or mesenteric occlusion (Bucy and Lesemann, 1942). Kalbag and Woolf (1967) documented a young man who developed raised intracranial pressure owing to sagittal sinus thrombosis and who died of liver failure a year later as a result of hepatic vein thrombosis.

The status of Buerger's disease is still uncertain, although it was described many years ago. It is said to be a rare inflammatory vasculitis affecting small and medium-sized arteries and veins occurring mostly in males under 40 years (Mills *et al.*, 1987). There is a strong association with cigarette smoking and a possible association with HLA types A9 and B5. Pathologically the characteristic features are focal segmental inflammatory infiltration affecting all vessel coats and combined with a cellular thrombus in the lumen. The inflammation is predominantly polymorphonuclear in the early stages, monocytic in the later stages and occasionally granulomatous with giant cells. The arterial intima is thickened, but there are no lipid deposits and the elastic lamina is intact. Evidence of recanalization is usually present within the organized thrombus and microabscesses are described occasionally.

The disease involves distal arteries of the limbs and often leads to peripheral gangrene and amputation. There is extensive arterial collateral development with a 'corkscrew' appearance on angiography. Recurrent venous thrombosis, often the first sign of the disease, may occur at any site but is commonest in the legs. Despite the histological evidence of inflammation, no infective or autoimmune process has been identified, and some regard Buerger's disease as primarily a thrombotic disorder, perhaps linked to hypersensitivity to tobacco or as the result of multiple arterial embolism.

A patient with typical Buerger's disease presenting as multiple venous sinus thrombosis in the brain has been seen (R. Ross Russell, unpublished observation).

IATROGENIC CEREBRAL VENOUS THROMBOSIS

Oral contraceptive drugs

The introduction of oral contraceptive drugs in the early 1960s was soon followed by reports of an increased incidence of venous thrombosis and thromboembolism. Oestrogens increase the risk of venous thrombosis and the risk is dose related. Large doses as used in the early trials on prostatic carcinoma and myocardial infarction caused a marked increase in death from pulmonary embolism but low-oestrogen preparations carry a relatively low risk. The mode of action is multifactorial; oestrogens increase the plasma concentration of fibrinogen and the coagulation Factors II, VII, VIII, IX and X. There is also depression of antithrombin III and reduced fibrinolytic activity in the vessel wall, all of which promote thrombosis. Other effects such as slowing of venous flow and endothelial damage may also be important. Within a few years it became apparent that there was also an increased risk of cerebral infarction from arterial occlusion, and that the risk was greatest in those with hypertension, diabetes or a history of heavy cigarette smoking.

Reports of intracranial venous thrombosis appeared later; Atkinson *et al.* (1970) described a young woman with aseptic thrombosis of the sagittal sinus, the right transverse sinus and the internal jugular vein occurring 2 months after starting oral contraceptives, and reviewed the literature on five similar cases. In some, multiple sinuses, including the cavernous sinus, were involved in a step-wise fashion. Thrombosis tended to occur shortly after starting the drug and to involve sinuses rather than cortical veins. Only one patient had seizures. Other early reports were from Buchanan and Brazinski (1970) and Fairburn (1973), and included a case successfully treated with anticoagulants. Estanol *et al.* (1979) found six patients on oral contraceptives out of a total of 20 young women with cerebral venous thrombosis in Brazil. A variety of sites were involved including the sphenoparietal sinus and the Galenic veins. They suggested that the rugose walls and trabeculation of the sinuses predisposed to platelet adhesion.

The finding by Bousser *et al.* (1985) of only three patients on oral contraceptives out of a total of 38 suggests that the low-oestrogen or progesterone preparations carry a much reduced risk. However, there has been recent concern over the safety of combined oral contraceptives containing third-generation progestogens. It now appears that this combination of drugs carries a greater risk of venous thromboembolism than the previous generation of oral contraceptives, and that the risk is especially high in carriers of the Factor V Leiden mutation and in those with a family history of thrombosis (Bloemenkamp *et al.*, 1995).

Other drug-induced thrombosis

There are many instances in the literature of patients developing venous thrombosis in the brain and elsewhere while on treatment with corticosteroids, but it is hard to know if thrombosis is attributable to the steroids or to the underlying condition for which the drug was given. The occasional occurrence of cerebral venous thrombosis in the course of Cushing's disease suggests that high corticosteroid levels may themselves be thrombogenic (R. Ross Russell, unpublished observation). Other types of steroid may also carry a similar risk. Hamed *et al.* (1989) reported two patients with intracranial hypertension and probable sagittal sinus thrombosis induced by danazol, an androgen derived from ethisterone used to treat endometriosis. It causes increased concentration of Factors VIII and IX, and kallikrein inhibitor. Androgens taken to enhance athletic performance have also led to cerebral venous sinus thrombosis in young healthy men (Jaillard *et al.*, 1994).

Cerebral venous thrombosis is also a potential hazard for patients receiving antifibrinolytic therapy for subarachnoid haemorrhage or for menorrhagia. Epsilon-aminocaproic acid acts by competitive inhibition of the activator converting plasminogen to plasmin and is thought to promote maturation of thrombus. A single case of sagittal sinus thrombosis in a patient receiving large doses of this drug was recorded by Ackiron *et al.* (1990).

L-Asparginase, an inhibitor of protein synthesis used in combination chemotherapy of acute lymphatic leukaemia is associated with a range of haemorrhagic and thrombotic complications owing to the interaction of procoagulant and anticoagulant proteins during the recovery phase (Steinherz *et al.*, 1981). Thromboses tend to occur later than haemorrhages after a latent interval of a few weeks. There is depletion of a number of plasma proteins including fibrinogen, Factors IX and XI, plasminogen, antithrombin III and proteins C and S. Cerebral venous thrombosis has also been reported following abuse of 'ecstasy', a stimulant drug containing amphetamine (Rothwell and Grant, 1993). Sumatriptan, recently introduced for the treatment of migraine, has been said to provoke stroke in patients already affected by sagittal sinus thrombosis (Cavazos *et al.*, 1994).

Venous cannulas

A different variety of iatrogenic thrombosis may result from the use of long-term venous cannulas placed in the brachial, subclavian or superior vena cava for post-operative fluid replacement or parenteral feeding, or sometimes misplaced inadvertently in the internal jugular vein. Thrombosis begins around the cannula and propagates back to the major venous sinuses causing raised intracranial pressure. Similar mishaps have followed delivery of toxic or hyperosmolar solutions (Souter and Mitchell, 1982), or after placement of a cardiac pacemaker (Floyd and Mahaley, 1969).

VENOUS THROMBOSIS SECONDARY TO DISTURBANCES IN FLOW

Physical factors causing stasis or slowing of blood flow predominate in this group of cerebral venous disorders. Stasis may be secondary to general dehydration or cardiac failure, or to local conditions such as branch artery occlusion or compression of a cerebral vein by tumour. The association between intracranial arteriovenous fistulas and venous thrombosis is being recognized with increasing frequency and is also included here.

DEHYDRATION

Dehydration is often cited as a factor predisposing to sino-venous thrombosis in the older literature, when describing the disease in infancy and childhood. Byers and Hass (1933) reporting 50 cases of the disease in infants under 2 years found only three with a clear infective origin; the remainder were acutely dehydrated with relative polycythaemia requiring intravenous fluid replacement. The underlying cause of the dehydration in most cases was fluid and electrolyte loss from diarrhoea and vomiting in the course of infantile gastroenteritis.

Any of the major venous sinuses may be involved; the mid-portion of the superior sagittal sinus has been cited as the most vulnerable area (Byers and Hass, 1933), and there are a number of reports of such children with thrombosis of the internal venous system including the straight sinus, the vein of Galen, the internal cerebral veins and the choroidal veins (Ehlers and Courville, 1936; Johnson *et al.*, 1973). Thrombosis may be widespread; it may involve more than one major sinus as well as cortical veins and there is often evidence of systemic venous thrombosis at autopsy.

The diagnosis of cerebral-venous thrombosis in such acutely ill and often malnourished infants is far from easy. Seizures are often the first indication of intracranial disease even in those cases where thrombosis involves the internal venous system, and other early features include raised intracranial pressure with headache, papilloedema, tonic spasms and bulging fontanelle. Unusual symptoms are pain in the teeth and jaws, trismus, and oedema of the eyelids and scalp. Distended scalp veins may be obvious on examination.

Even in more recent times dehydration remains an important factor in the neonatal period. Barron *et al.* (1992) make a distinction between the disease in neonates and in older children. In neonates they found 80% presenting with seizures in a setting of acute systemic illness, hypotension and dehydration; this group has a poor prognosis. By contrast in older children the presenting symptom is usually headache and the underlying cause a prothrombotic state or an infection.

Dehydration again becomes important at the other extreme of life in the course of wasting or malignant disease, particularly where there is dysphagia or impairment of consciousness, and where fluid and electrolyte replacement has been inadequate (Barnett and Hyland, 1953). In middle life, dehydration and relative polycythaemia seldom become severe enough to cause thrombosis from impairment of blood flow in the veins, but Ata (1965) described two fatal cases in association with severe diabetic coma and hypotension. In one the internal jugular vein was thrombosed, and there was infarction of the cerebellum and brainstem. There was also pituitary infarction. Another unusual instance of thrombosis of the straight sinus causing bilateral cerebellar infarction has been reported recently in an adult diabetic patient with severe hyperosmolar coma (Eng *et al.*, 1990).

OBSTRUCTIVE LESIONS OF THE DURAL SINUSES

Surgeons in the last century were well aware that ligation of the internal jugular vein in the course of operations on tuberculous glands or in block dissection of the neck was occasionally followed by raised intracranial pressure, and that this was more likely to occur after ligation of the right side, which normally drains the superior sagittal sinus (Bradshaw, 1956). Many of these patients showed the syndrome of 'benign intracranial hypertension' without cerebral infarction and even a narrowing of the vein at the jugular foramen may be sufficient to raise the intracranial pressure (Mones, 1965). Locally invasive tumours such as carcinoma of the parotid gland are likely in addition to cause thrombosis of the vein, which may then propagate to the lateral sinus and torcula, eventually resulting in cerebral infarction (Tourbin, 1973).

Partial or complete obstruction to blood flow in any of the major sinuses may occur as a result of external compression by tumour, overgrowth or displacement of adjacent bone, or from mass lesions within the sinus itself. The effects depend on the site of obstruction and on the rate of occlusion, and are discussed later. In the superior sagittal sinus even partial obstruction is capable of causing interference to absorption of CSF and consequent intracranial hypertension. This is well illustrated in a remarkable case history published by Caudill *et al.* (1953). The patient had a posterior parietal depressed skull fracture producing raised intracranial pressure but without thrombosis of the sinus. The raised pressure in the sinus and in the CSF was immediately relieved by elevation of the skull fracture.

OBSTRUCTION BY TUMOUR

Any of the major venous sinues may be blocked by a local tumour deposit, either a primary tumour such as meningioma, glomus tumour or sarcoma of the skull vault or a metastatic lesion. Blockage of the sinuses is more likely to occur when the malignant process involves the meninges rather than the skull vault. Clinical effects are likely only in the case of the superior sagittal sinus, lateral sinus or occasionally in jugular vein occlusion when intracranial hypertension may occur (Enevoldson and Ross Russell, 1990). Sigsbee *et al.* (1979) reviewed 14 patients of this kind. In 12 the primary tumour was solid and in 2 it was haematogenous. Carcinoma of the breast or cervix was a common primary site and, in the haematogenous group, acute lymphocytic and monocytic leukaemia predominated. Sagittal sinus thrombosis has been recorded at the site of a metastasis of a carcinoid tumour by Patchell and Posner (1986). In children, increased intracranial pressure as a result of blockage of the sagittal sinus by secondary neuroblastoma has also been reported (Mones, 1965) as has subarachnoid spread of a medulloblastoma (Brown *et al.*, 1991).

In patients undergoing treatment for advanced malignant disease, sinus thrombosis tends to happen either during chemotherapy or in the terminal stages of the illness. At autopsy narrowing or occlusion of the sinus and infiltration of the walls with tumour or leukaemic cells has been demonstrated (Mones, 1965). Nine patients with metastatic disease from Ewing's sarcoma or from plasmocytoma producing a complete or partial occlusion of the superior sagittal sinus were described by Plant *et al.* (1991). They found an extradural tissue mass beneath the inner table of the skull, which distorted or compressed the sinus but did not necessarily cause thrombosis. The patients presented with raised intracranial pressure and in some the pressure returned to normal after surgical removal of the lesion. Because obstruction usually takes place slowly, collateral venous pathways, including scalp veins, are prominent and, although intracranial pressure may be increased, there may be no thrombosis of the sinus and no venous infarction of the brain. In one case quoted by Plant *et al.* (1991), the sagittal sinus was partially occluded in its posterior third by a mass of extradural plasmocytoma lying beneath the inner table of the skull. Intracranial hypertension was relieved following removal of the tumour.

Glomus tumours are a special case, since they originate in remnants of chromaffin tissue in close relation to the jugular foramen and middle ear, and may actually invade the lumen of the internal jugular vein causing obstruction and sometimes a spreading thrombosis. Examples of right-sided or bilateral glomus tumours causing intracranial hypertension are quoted by Kalbag and Woolf (1967) and by Enevoldson and Ross Russell (1990).

Meningioma arising in relation to the walls of the dural sinuses is also liable to cause obstruction of the sinus as an early feature. Meningioma of this type may arise in the groove of the sigmoid sinus (Yokota *et al.*, 1993) or in the falco-tentorial region obstructing the straight sinus (Odake, 1992).

SINO-VENOUS THROMBOSIS SECONDARY TO ARTERIAL OCCLUSION

Observations on the pial vasculature during experimental arterial occlusion have described changes in the veins as an early event. The blood flow in small veins is visibly slowed and the blood appears granular as a result of rouleux formation with aggregation of red cells. White platelet thrombi form in the small venules; they adhere to the endothelium for a time, then break off and are carried towards larger veins and the sagittal sinus. Mixed or red venous thrombi are not seen (Ross Russell 1966). When blood flow is very slow, the clumps of cells may be separated from each other by clear zones of plasma (cattle-trucking) and, under conditions of near stagnation, the cellular elements may remain impacted, permitting passage of plasma only (plasma skimming). The rheological properties of blood are altered under conditions of slow flow and there is a marked increase in whole-blood viscosity. It is suggested that adhesion of platelets to the walls of small venules is a result of anoxic damage to the endothelium.

In spite of these observations and the fact that clinical arterial occlusion in man must cause a similar retardation of blood flow in cerebral veins, there are few descriptions of venous thrombosis as a consequence of arterial occlusion. Noetzel and Jerusalem (1965) quote arteriosclerosis and hypertension as the underlying cause of sino-venous thrombosis in 19 out of 105 patients, but it is not clear how many of these had suffered a cerebral arterial thrombosis. Barnett and Hyland (1953) in a pathological study of 39 cases found three examples of ante-mortem thrombosis of cortical veins or venous sinuses that followed thrombosis of a major cerebral artery. There was also one instance of sagittal sinus thrombosis following a hypertensive cerebral haemorrhage. Two further cases were reported by Kalbag and Woolf (1967) following infarction in the middle cerebral artery territory. In one, histological examination indicated that the venous thrombosis occurred considerably later than the arterial event.

The converse, with arterial occlusion occurring as a consequence of venous thrombosis, may be seen in the cavernous sinus where the internal carotid artery is enveloped by the venous sinus. This is most likely to occur in infective thrombosis (Sekhar *et al.*, 1980).

In summary, although thrombosis of cortical veins is probably not uncommon overlying an acute cerebral infarct, it has no influence on the evolution of the lesion provided that it does not spread to the major sinuses. The development of signs of raised intracranial pressure at an interval after arterial infarction should raise the possibility of sagittal sinus thrombosis (Barnett and Hyland, 1953).

HEART DISEASE

'The state of the circulation' was one of the principal factors in the pathogenesis of primary venous thrombosis, according to Gowers (1893) who described sagittal sinus thrombosis occurring in the very old and the very young. Congestive cardiac failure is a well-recognized forerunner of deep vein thrombosis in the legs, and its importance in the cerebral circulation was emphasized by Barnett and Hyland (1953) who reviewed 39 cases of non-infective intracranial venous thrombosis coming to autopsy in a general hospital.

Cardiac failure was the only recognizable cause in ten patients. In most cases there was haemorrhagic infarction secondary to occlusion of superficial or deep cerebral veins; in only a minority was there occlusion of the dural sinuses. In three patients the venous thrombosis appeared to be the cause of death, in four it was a contributory factor and in three (without cerebral infarction) the vein thrombosis was probably the terminal event. The patients were elderly, emaciated or dehydrated, and five had advanced carcinomatosis. The cardiac failure was of recent onset and was mainly right-sided and severe. There were also five cases of post-operative venous thrombosis, mostly following abdominal operations and cerebral thrombosis was the cause of death in four of these. One patient had both arterial and venous cerebral thrombosis in the same region of the brain. Histological examination of the veins showed evidence of thrombosis of varying ages, which appeared to have originated *in situ*, and some of these patients had shown ingravescent or intermittent symptoms during life.

Similar instances of latent cerebral venous infarction affecting the sinuses rather than the superficial veins were reported by Towbin (1973). There were 17 cases in 182 autopsies of elderly subjects; most were women with signs of cardiac failure dehydration or emaciation. Thromboembolic events in other sites were commonplace, especially pulmonary embolism. The symptomatology in these cases was of lethargy progressing to coma without fever, meningeal or focal cerebral signs. The brain showed patchy or confluent neuronal loss mainly affecting cortical layers 3 and 5 with scattered haemorrhagic infarction. Transverse, sigmoid or sagittal sinuses were thrombosed.

It is evident from these reports that venous or dural sinus thrombosis occurs much more frequently than official statistics suggest (reported deaths from cerebral venous thrombosis in UK were approximately 20 per year in the 1970s). It is not unusual as a terminal event and many cases must escape detection. There is unlikely to be a single cause but slowing of the circulation as a result of cardiac failure may well be an important factor, although not the only one. Experimental work has shown the difficulty of inducing venous thrombosis by ligation alone. There is a large area of overlap with the prothrombotic states seen in many types of malignant disease, many of which, including disseminated intravascular coagulation, may be clinically unsuspected (Kim *et al.*, 1976).

ARTERIOVENOUS MALFORMATION

Dural arteriovenous fistulas are tangles of dilated thin-walled veins and small arteries usually derived from dural and meningeal branches of the external carotid system. At some point there is a direct communication between arteries and veins leading to an abnormally high pressure and flow in the veins with progressive enlargement. Feeding arteries, which are often derived from a number of the major vessels, also become hypertrophied in response to an increased flow.

This type of malformation occurs mainly in relation to the major venous sinuses at the base of the skull. There are two groups; an anterio-inferior group related to the cavernous, sphenoparietal and petrosal sinuses, and a superioposterior group related to the sagittal, straight, transverse, sigmoid and occipital sinuses (Aminoff, 1973). The origin of these lesions is uncertain but they may be acquired rather than congenital, and they may show progressive enlargement. There is a tendency to spontaneous cure.

Presentation is usually in middle age with symptoms of venous hypertension affecting either the cavernous, transverse, or sagittal sinus. Other symptoms are pulsatile tinnitus, seizures, or venous infarction affecting the hemispheres or cerebellum. There is also some risk of haemorrhage.

It has now been well established that there is an association between dural arterio-venous malformations and thrombosis of adjacent veins or sinuses, but it is still not clear whether the malformation causes the thrombosis or vice versa. Microscopic examination of excised specimens of malformations shows a mass of dilated blood vessels sometimes with characteristics of a cavernous angioma but it does not allow definite conclusions on the origin of these lesions. The development of the malformation has been demonstrated radiologically over a period of years after occlusion of a major sinus (Houser *et al.*, 1979). It has been suggested that, during the process of organization of a sinus thrombus, small dural arterioles may rupture into the lumen of the vein, thus initiating a fistulous communication between the arterial and venous systems, which then progressively enlarges as new feeding vessels develop. Trauma has also been held responsible, as in other types of arterio-venous fistula (Hayes, 1963).

On the other hand there are examples of venous and sinus thrombosis occurring in patients with established dural malformation and this may be a way by which the lesions sometimes undergo spontaneous cure. It is not easy to explain why a dural arterio-venous malformation should cause thrombosis of a neighbouring dural sinus, but it may be that the abnormally high venous pressure and flow associated with a fistula causes endothelial damage to the draining vein or sinus with resultant thrombosis (Enevoldson and Ross Russell, 1990). Examples of arterio-venous malformations presenting as isolated intracranial hypertension are quoted by Tajima *et al.* (1991) and by Jacewicz and Plum (1990), as cortical venous infarction by Mineta *et al.* (1991), as pulsatile tinnitus and focal deficit by Houser *et al.* (1979), and as cavernous sinus syndrome by Brunquell and Rosenberger (1982). Nakahara *et al.* (1993) in an authoritative report described five adult patients with posterior fossa dural arteriovenous fistulas who showed an 'isolated sinus segment' caused by sinus thrombosis. The malformations were situated at the transverse sigmoid sinus (three cases), superior petrosal sinus (one case) and straight sinus (one case), and were fed by many branches of the external carotid artery, including the middle meningeal, ascending pharyngeal, posterior auricular and occipital. Meningeal branches of the vertebral or posterior cerebral arteries and the meningo-hypophyseal branch of the internal carotid artery also contributed. Venous drainage of the malformations was via the isolated sinus segment to the contralateral transverse or supratentorial sinuses through markedly dilated cortical or deep venous collaterals. A single patient with thrombosis of the deep cerebral veins associated with an extensive medullary venous malformation was described by Abumiya *et al.* (1992). Fibrinolytic treatment was followed by partial recanalization of the veins and disappearance of the malformation. The authors suggest that the venous thrombosis was the primary event and was followed by abnormal venous drainage via persistent embryonic vessels.

Although in the majority of patients with venous thrombosis of this type the arterio-venous malformation is situated in the dura, there are also instances of intracerebral malformations with the same complication (Figure 4.1). These are usually in the cerebral hemispheres at a short distance from the sagittal sinus; they are not necessarily visible on the surface of the brain but enlarged draining veins may be seen (Waggoner, 1928) and the distension as a result of increased pressure may extend to dural sinuses at some distance from the malformation. The effects usually depend on the size and behaviour of the malformation and on the occurrence of haemorrhage, but thrombosis of a draining vein may give rise to a venous infarct either in the superficial or deep venous territories or to intracranial hypertension (Enevoldson and Ross Russell, 1990). In the case of the cavernous sinus, which may be distended with arterialized blood causing proptosis and ophthalmoplegia, the occurrence of venous thrombosis may bring about a spontaneous cure.

SINUS AND VENOUS THROMBOSIS CAUSED BY MENINGEAL INFECTION OR INFILTRATION

A meningeal inflammatory reaction, either infective or non-infective, spreading to the walls of arteries and veins on the surface of the brain may lead not only

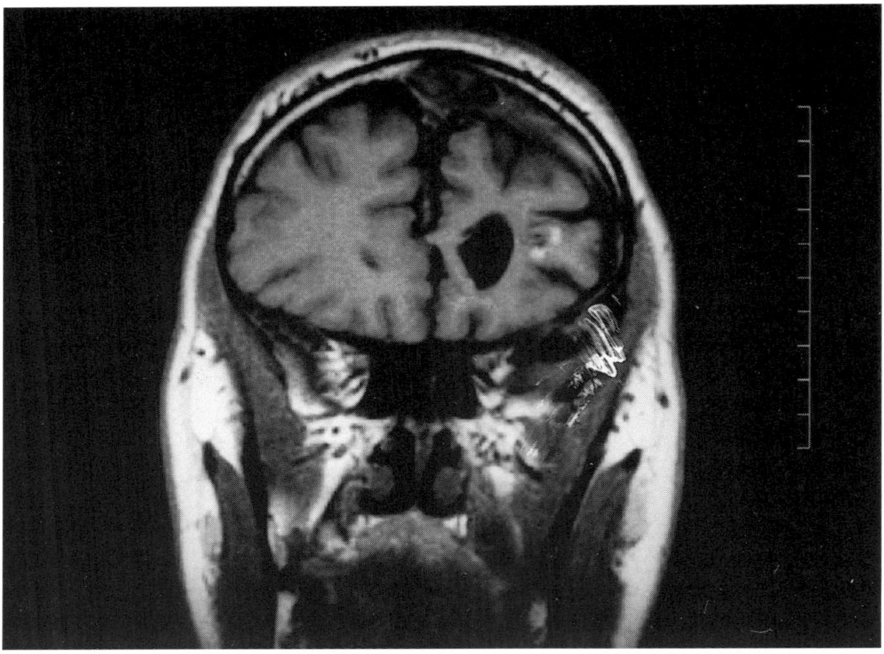

Figure 4.1 Thrombosis of the superior sagittal sinus in a patient with an intracerebral arteriovenous malformation. The thrombus shows evidence of organization and recanalization.

to a narrowing of the vessels, but also to intravascular thrombosis. Otitic bacterial infections, once the predominant cause of cerebral venous thrombosis, have been succeeded by other types of infection with obscure or resistant organisms. Also included in this group are a number of unusual meningeal infiltrations, granulomatous or neoplastic, which may involve the walls of cerebral veins or sinuses.

INFECTIVE THROMBOSIS

In the pre-antibiotic era, infection was much the commonest cause of thrombosis of the venous sinuses (Gowers, 1893). Even in 1956 it accounted for 60% of the 42 patients with sinus thrombosis reported by Bradshaw, but it is now rarely seen. The infection may originate in the upper respiratory tract, the skin, the bone or the meninges, and there may be an associated cerebral abscess. The emissary veins of the skull may provide a route for a surface infection to reach the cerebral venous system. The venous sinuses most often involved are the lateral sinus, the cavernous sinus and the superior sagittal sinus.

Infective Lateral Sinus Thrombosis

Lateral sinus thrombosis is usually a sequel of bacterial infection of the middle ear and mastoid, and affects debilitated children. It may occur either in the acute or the chronic stages of the illness and the responsible organism is most often a beta-haemolytic streptococcus. A septicaemia is present in about 50% of cases. The onset of lateral sinus thrombosis is accompanied by a worsening of fever and rigors, and by headache, nausea and vomiting. Local signs of inflammation are usually absent but there may be swelling over the mastoid region, distension of the superficial veins and tenderness over the jugular vein (Kinal and Jaeger, 1960). Raised intracranial pressure occurs in about half the cases and is more common when the right side is involved; it signifies spread of thrombosis to the torcular and superior sagittal sinus and is shown by drowsiness and bilateral papilloedema, and by separation of the sutures and bulging fontanelle in infants. Unilateral papilloedema, proptosis or ophthalmoplegia suggests extension of thrombosis to the cavernous sinus. The occurrence of focal or generalized seizures suggests spread of thrombosis to cortical or anastomotic veins, or the development of a cerebral abscess. Other features are an abducens palsy signifying either raised intracranial pressure or thrombosis of the inferior petrosal sinus. There may also be ipsilateral facial pain from spread of infection to the petrous apex and adjacent Gasserian ganglion. Involvement of lower cranial nerves (ninth, tenth and eleventh) is unusual, but may occur from local osteomyelitis or thrombosis of the sigmoid sinus and jugular vein.

Infective thrombosis of the sigmoid and lateral sinus was reviewed by Reading and Schurr (1956) in relation to the introduction of antibiotics. In the days before sulphonamides, acute mastoiditis was a common illness and the prevalence of sinus thrombosis was 1.9%. In the sulphonamide era, there were many fewer cases but the prevalence of sinus thrombosis in these patients remained unchanged. The introduction of penicillin reduced the frequency of acute mastoiditis still further, but in patients with chronic mastoid infection with bone erosion or cholesteatoma formation, sinus thrombosis was still seen in about 5–10% of cases. Such patients tended to run a relapsing course with a low fever and a poor response to antibiotics. The infecting organism is now most commonly *Proteus*, *E. coli* or anaerobes.

Thrombosis of the sigmoid and lateral sinus may be followed by resorption and recanalisation, by embolization of a fragment of infected thrombus to the lungs leading to generalized pyaemia, or by retrograde extension of the thrombus to the other intracranial veins and sinuses. Reading and Schurr (1956) reported that thrombosis extended into the jugular vein in 20% of patients. The mortality, which was 25% in the pre-antibiotic era, was caused by cerebral abscess, meningitis or pyaemia. At one time ligation of the jugular vein was recommended to prevent embolization of infected thrombus (Bradshaw, 1956); exposure and incision of the sigmoid sinus with thrombectomy was also practised (Reading and Schurr, 1956). At the present time in developed countries, acute mastoiditis has almost disappeared but chronic mastoiditis still occurs, and may present as sinus thrombosis or intracranial hypertension with little evidence of infection [otitic hydrocephalus of Symonds (1937)]. A region of sterile granulation tissue may be discovered adjacent to the thrombosed sinus (Williams and Richardson, 1988).

Infective Cavernous Sinus Thrombosis

Thrombosis of the cavernous sinus is caused almost exclusively by infection and has now almost disappeared in developed countries except in patients with a compromised immune system, with diabetes, leukaemia or steroid treatment. Infections with resistant or unusual organisms, such as mucormycosis or *Aspergillus* have become more common. Formerly cavernous sinus thrombosis followed regional infection with *Staphylococcus aureus, Streptococcus pneumoniae, Haemophilus influenzae* or anaerobes, and the mortality approached 100% from septicaemia and meningitis. Even with modern antibiotic treatment, the mortality is still approximately 30%. The site of infection is often the skin of the upper face or scalp, the orbit or the upper respiratory tract, and the route of infection the orbital and pterygoid veins. In recent years, infection originating in the sphenoid or ethmoid sinus has become the commonest source of infection (Southwick *et al.*, 1986). The infecting organism has also changed; agents, such as *Aspergillus*, are now the commonest cause, especially in immunocompromised patients or those receiving steroids (Sekhar *et al.*, 1980).

Sometimes infection may follow trauma or surgery. Anterior and posterior varieties are described depending on the source of infection (Brown, 1961). There may be spread from the middle ear and mastoid region via the sigmoid sinus and petrosal sinus (Symonds, 1937). This variety tends to run a more chronic course.

Infective thrombosis begins on one side; it may spread to the other by the circular sinus but with improvements in treatment unilateral cases are now as common as bilateral. There may also be spread to the pituitary with necrosis of the gland and the cavernous portion of the internal carotid artery may be involved. The cavernous sinus receives additional tributaries from the cortical venous system via the middle and inferior superficial cerebral veins. Infection may propagate via these routes to cause cerebral abscess, subdural empyema or meningitis; there is frequently a CSF pleocytosis.

Infective Sagittal Sinus Thrombosis

Infection is an uncommon cause of thrombosis in this situation; a few examples may be found from the days before antibiotics as a complication of osteomyelitis of the skull vault or from frontal, maxillary or ethmoidal sinusitis (Doyle, 1927). Infection may also be a contributory factor in traumatic lesions involving the vertex of the skull and in cases of meningitis. The responsible organisms may be *S. pneumoniae, Staph. aureus* or *Haemophilus* (Southwick *et al.*, 1986). Sagittal sinus thrombosis may also occur as a result of spread of infected thrombus from the lateral sinuses in otitic infections.

The onset of sagittal sinus thrombosis is marked by a rapid deterioration in the condition of the patient, a decline in the level of consciousness, unilateral or bilateral hemiparesis, or seizures. Headache, vomiting and swinging pyrexia are prominent, and the CSF usually but not invariably shows inflammatory cells. Signs of raised intracranial pressure with papilloedema develop later but may not be obvious at an early stage. There may be indications of raised venous pressure, such as oedema of the eyelids, and distension of small veins on the eyelids and forehead (Doyle, 1927). Infective thrombosis of the sagittal sinus was formerly almost uniformly fatal and still carries a substantial mortality approaching 80%.

Cortical Vein Thrombosis

Septic thrombosis of superficial cortical veins may occur in the course of meningeal infections, usually accompanied by spread to the sagittal sinus. In an autopsy series, the prevalence of cortical vein thrombophlebitis was 5% (DiNubile *et al.*, 1990) but the diagnosis was documented in life in only 1% of 790 cases of bacterial meningitis in Boston in 1960–1984. The commonest infecting organism is *Streptococcus pneumoniae* and the clinical signs included fever, seizures and focal neurological deficits. Half the patients survived but the majority of these had persisting disability. In the autopsy series other pathological processes such as arteritis, cerebral infarction and ventriculitis were more prominent than thrombophlebitis (DiNubile *et al.*, 1990). It appears that septic cortical venous thrombosis may be less important as a cause of seizures and focal neurological deficit than was once thought.

Infections of other kinds involving the meninges have occasionally occurred with sinus or venous thrombosis. An adult case of trichinosis with meningoencephalitis and sinus thrombosis has been reported (Evans and Patten, 1982). Venous thrombosis with virus infections of the brain appears to be exceptionally rare but a single case of *Cytomegalovirus* meningoencephalitis causing sagittal sinus occlusion in a young human immunodeficiency virus (HIV)-positive woman is on record (Meyohas *et al.*, 1989).

WEGENER'S GRANULOMATOSIS

This variety of pulmonary granulomatous vasculitis combines lesions of the upper and lower respiratory tract with a focal necrotizing glomerulo-nephritis. It usually presents in middle-aged men with cough, chest pain or haemoptysis accompanied by nasal granulomas and epistaxis. Renal involvement can be asymptomatic or acute. Other features are malaise, fever and arthralgia. Neurological complications take the form of uveitis, orbital pseudotumour and polyneuropathy. The typical histological changes are best seen in the lungs and consist of nodules of histiocytes, plasma cells and lymphocytes with giant cells and central necrosis. Normocytic anaemia, raised erythrocyte sedimentation rate (ESR) are the rule and the most reliable immunological abnormality is a raised titre of antineutrophilic cytoplasmic antibody (ANCA).

Brain lesions in Wegener's granuloma are rare; there may be typical granulomas within the cerebral substance surrounded by vasculitis in small arteries and veins. Reports have appeared of large necrotic lesions of the frontal lobe caused by necrotizing thrombophlebitis with occlusion of the superior sagittal sinus (Mickle *et al.*, 1977), and of a meningeal granulomatous process causing sagittal sinus thrombosis and raised intracranial pressure (Enevoldson and Ross Russell, 1990).

BEHÇET'S SYNDROME

The original descriptions of this syndrome were of a chronic relapsing oro-genital ulceration with uveitis. More recently, a number of other features have been added, notably skin rash (erythema nodosum), arthritis, and neurological and vascular lesions, usually venous. The cause is unknown, but there is strong evidence for an immunological abnormality and a link with HLA types. HLA-B51 is significantly associated with the disease in some parts of the world, and this and other antigens are also concerned with tissue localization. HLA-DR7 is strongly associated with ocular and neurological lesions.

Pathologically there is early lymphocytic infiltration of the lamina propria, epithelium and small vessels in the neighbourhood of the lesions, with endothelial proliferation and narrowing of vessels, especially veins. Circulating immune complexes have been detected by various methods in 40–60% of patients. Acute-phase proteins, notably C-reactive protein and C9, are increased.

The disease is particularly common in Japan and in the Middle East, and usually affects males in the third decade. Behçets syndrome was the commonest cause of cerebral venous thrombosis in the series of 40 patients reported from Saudi Arabia by Daif *et al.* (1995). Neurological involvement occurs in 10–25% of patients in the form of a relapsing meningo-encephalitis with a marked lymphocytic reaction in the cerebrospinal fluid. Focal lesions may occur, most often in the brainstem or spinal cord. Although thrombophlebitis is a recognized feature of the disease in about one quarter of patients and affecting veins at any site, including the superior vena cava, there appears to be a particular tendency to involve the cerebral venous sinuses. This was first described by Masheter (1959) and confirmed in many recent reports (Kozin *et al.*, 1977; Bousser *et al.*, 1980; Pamir *et al.*, 1981; Bousser *et al.*, 1985; Wechster *et al.*, 1992). It is claimed that as many as 40% of patients with neurological features have superior sagittal sinus thrombosis (Bank and Weart, 1984), often with no signs of thrombosis elsewhere. The usual mode of presentation is as raised intracranial pressure with headache and papilloedema occurring after symptoms have been present for several months. The two patients reported by Kozin *et al.* (1977) had swelling of the basal ganglia, presumably oedema or infarction as a result of internal cerebral vein occlusion.

Some patients recover spontaneously or after repeated lumbar puncture, but most now receive corticosteroids, immunosuppressive or immunopotentiating therapy, or colchicine. Anticoagulants have been recommended but the occurrence of pulmonary arterial aneurysms in some cases has limited this form of treatment.

SARCOIDOSIS

Approximately 5% of patients with sarcoidosis have neurological involvement, usually in the form of a granulomatous meningeal reaction causing cranial nerve palsies or hydrocephalus from fourth ventricle outflow obstruction. The protein content of the cerebrospinal fluid is markedly increased. Sarcoid lesions of the cerebral parenchyma are much less common, and tend to affect the hypothalamic and pituitary region. The majority of patients have features of systemic sarcoidosis, usually in the lungs, lymph nodes, uveal tract or skin, but isolated neurological sarcoidosis is well recognized. The diagnosis is usually made by biopsy of an affected gland or by a positive granulomatous reaction to intradermal Kveim antigen. Increased uptake of gallium-67 by parotid, lacrimal glands or mediastinum is strong supporting evidence.

Thrombosis of venous sinuses has been reported but, because sarcoidosis affects mainly the basal meninges, the sagittal sinus is not often involved. A well-documented patient, a West Indian man aged 32 with a protracted illness causing intracranial hypertension, was described by Byrne and Lawton (1983). There was narrowing of the right lateral sinus and the left did not fill at all. The vein of Galen was abnormally small and drained by a network of small venous collaterals in the occipital region. Computed tomography (CT) scanning showed intense dural enhancement of the falx and tentorium cerebelli, and the vein of Galen (an inconstant feature of sarcoidosis). The diagnosis was made by meningeal biopsy. A further patient with ocular sarcoid but no previous neurological lesion developed intracranial hypertension secondary to dural sinus thrombosis, and made a good recovery on corticosteroid treatment (Akova *et al.*, 1993).

LYMPHOMA

Intracerebral deposits of lymphoma are unusual in Hodgkin's disease, although compression of the spinal cord is not uncommon. In non-Hodgkin's lymphoma, however, lymphomatous masses may occur in the orbit or intracranially either as a meningeal infiltrate or as discrete deposits within the cerebral substance. Immunocompromised patients, either as a result of HIV infection or from immunosuppressive treatment, are at particular risk.

Occasional examples of malignant lymphoma occurring in association with cerebral venous thrombosis can be found in papers quoting large series of cases (Bousser *et al.*, 1985). Of the eight cases of cerebral venous thrombosis associated with lymphoproliferative diseases quoted by Meininger *et al.* (1985), five had acute lymphoblastic leukaemia and three had non-Hodgkin's lymphoma. The superior sagittal sinus was involved in all but one case. As with many of the cases of sinus thrombosis occurring with malignant disease, it is difficult to separate the effects of the disease from the side-effects of treatment and there is a suspicion that intrathecal methotrexate may be partly responsible.

The most detailed case report is of a 59-year-old man with lymphoma causing spinal compression, who developed sudden aphasia and right hemiparesis, and was found to have multiple regions of haemorrhagic cerebral and cerebellar infarction. At autopsy the walls of cerebral parenchymal and meningeal veins were found to be extensively infiltrated with lymphoma cells, and these were also present within the lumen of veins and capillaries causing leukostasis. The large dural sinuses were unaffected and veins elsewhere in the body were normal (Azzarelli *et al.*, 1980).

OTHER MISCELLANEOUS CAUSES OF CEREBRAL VENOUS THROMBOSIS

TRAUMATIC THROMBOSIS

Direct injury to the superior sagittal sinus occurred not infrequently in the days of trench warfare in World War I as a result of tangential gunshot wounds to the skull vertex. There was always extensive associated damage to the scalp and frequently (though not invariably) a gutter-like depressed fracture of the frontal or parietal bones. Injury to the large parietal lacunae, which receive the Rolandic veins draining the pre- and post-central gyri, led to thrombosis, which then propagated to the sagittal sinus or retrogradely to the cortical veins. In addition to venous infarction, there was a variable amount of local cerebral contusion and haemorrhage.

Holmes and Sargent published a classical account of 70 patients with such injuries in 1915, describing the characteristic neurological deficit produced by thrombosis of the sagittal sinus in the posterior frontal region combined with Rolandic vein thrombosis on one or both sides. The injured patients showed unilateral or bilateral hemiparesis markedly worse in the leg than the arm and with an early form of hypertonus, which resembled rigidity rather than classical spasticity, and produced adduction and inward rotation of the leg. Weakness affected the distal rather than the proximal part of the leg and the hand often retained normal power. The trunk, including the paraspinal muscles, was sometimes included in the hemiplegia. Speech, face and tongue were spared. The leg often showed a marked sensory ataxia and astereognosis with loss of joint position sense and two-point discrimination. Voluntary saccadic ocular movements were impaired but smooth pursuit was preserved. Seizures were a feature of some cases and retention of urine occurred occasionally. Confirmation of cerebral venous thrombosis was obtained at autopsy in those patients with severe associated brain injury, but Holmes and Sargent also recorded good recovery in some patients.

Barker (1949) published his findings in a group of similar patients wounded in World War II and showing signs of damage to the sagittal sinus. Four out of 11 patients had no loss of consciousness at the time of injury; all had severe tangential scalp laceration and seven had a depressed fracture. The syndrome of unilateral or bilateral crural monoplegia described previously was confirmed, and almost all patients had prominent sensory loss of cortical type affecting proprioception and tactile localization. He also noted the early appearance of hypertonus immediately after injury without any early flaccid stage. Headache and epilepsy were rare occurrences, although follow-up extended over some years. The injuries were consistent with venous infarction of the superior parts of the pre- and post-central gyri produced by thrombosis of the parietal lacuna, and the sagittal sinus which receives the Rolandic veins.

In more recent times, road traffic accidents have been responsible for most venous complications of skull trauma. Direct damage to the transverse or sigmoid sinus or to the torcular may follow fractures of the skull in the occipital area. Ecker (1946) described 11 such patients in which the fracture line crossed a venous sinus. In some, the blood flow in the sinus continued uninterrupted but in most cases there was local thrombosis at the fracture site followed by signs of raised intracranial pressure. Caudill *et al.* (1953) described a patient with a depressed fracture in the posterior parietal region, causing raised intracranial pressure from partial obstruction of venous drainage but without thrombosis of the sinus. Symptoms were relieved and intracranial pressure reduced after elevation of the fracture. In the 14 cases described by Kinal (1967) thrombosis was shown to extend by propagation as far as the torcular with consequent increased collateral flow via diploic and scalp veins, and the vertebral plexus. In children with craniosynostosis, in whom the jugular foramen may be narrowed be bony overgrowth, the cerebral venous drainage may be critically dependent on these collateral pathways. If these are divided during surgical attempts at skull reconstruction, raised intracranial pressure may result. In general, the course of traumatic sinus occlusion is benign; most patients do not develop venous infarction and raised intracranial pressure subsides as collateral channels develop.

The cranial sinuses may also thrombose after severe or sometimes minor closed head injury. This important condition was first described well in five patients by Martin (1955) and named traumatic hydrocephalus, although there was no ventricular dilatation. There was usually a 10-day interval between injury and evidence of brain damage during which time thrombus spread from scalp veins via diploic veins to the intracranial lacunae and major sinuses. Two clinical syndromes were described according to the extent of spread: the first being intracranial hypertension and abducens palsy caused by obstruction to CSF absorption, and the second a crural monoplegia similar to that documented by Holmes and Sargent 40 years earlier (1915).

CEREBRAL VENOUS DISEASE IN INFANCY AND CHILDHOOD

A century ago cerebral venous thrombosis was a frequent finding at autopsy of small children: Lidell's paper in 1874 was based on no less than 128 cases. Even in more recent times, 29 of the 105 patients described by Noetzel and Jerusalem (1965) were infants. They fall into the two main categories suggested by Gowers (1893), those secondary to the state of the circulation and those caused by local disease. The first group included infants, usually under 2 years old with severe dehydration from diarrhoea and vomiting, as well as malnourished and cachectic infants suffering from systemic disease or neglect. Cyanotic congenital heart disease is also a predisposing feature. Cerebral venous thrombosis was mainly a terminal event and was frequently undiagnosed during life. The sagittal sinus was most often involved, but thrombosis could be widespread including both superficial and deep venous sytems. Histological examination showed no evidence of inflammation in the vessel wall.

The second major group, those secondary to infection, included many examples of otitis media and meningitis, both acute and chronic, in which surface veins, arteries and cranial nerves were surrounded by inflammatory exudate and the venous walls were infiltrated with leucocytes. As the importance of infection as a cause of thrombosis has declined in recent years, increasing numbers of children with prothrombotic states have been recognized (Barron *et al.*, 1992).

The pathological changes in the brain in venous infarction differ in children and adults. Banker (1961) described three principal types. In the first type, mainly children with cyanotic heart disease, thrombus was present in the jugular veins, spreading to involve the sagittal sinus, cortical veins and sometimes the Galenic system. There were multiple infarcts in cortex and white matter, notably fronto-parietal in distribution. Histologically the infarcted tissue was filled with macrophages, astrocytes and activated microglia with distension and proliferation of small blood vessels and areas of haemorrhage.

A second type of pathological response was infarction in the territory of the internal cerebral veins, chiefly the globus pallidus and thalamus. A prominent histological feature, peculiar to infant and young children, was the finding of club-like processes representing interrupted axis cylinders.

The third type of pathological response was seen in infants dying shortly after birth and found to have a diffuse periventricular leucoencephalopathy, possibly developing *in utero*, in the distribution of the Galenic veins. This consisted of foci of necrotic white matter surrounding distended veins with a similar pattern of reactive astrocytes, microglia and degenerating axis cylinders. The diagnosis of venous occlusive disease was inferred in some cases from the distribution of lesions. Veins themselves were not always occluded, some showing recanalization and some being normal.

Byers and Hass (1933) published a review of 50 cases. In children under 2 years old, 'primary' cases predominated including many examples of dehydration and relative polycythaemia. In secondary (infective) cases, there were instances of infection with *Haemophilus influenzae, Strep. pneumoniae, E. coli* and *Mycobacterium tuberculosis*. They described some unusual clinical features in the primary group. In addition to seizures and features of raised intracranial pressure, there were examples of scalp and eyelid oedema and enlargement of scalp veins. In neonates, seizures, macroencephaly and respiratory depression may be presenting features (Grossman *et al.*, 1993).

The most comprehensive recent review of venous thrombosis in children was published from Philadelphia by Barron *et al.* (1992). The different modes of presentation and outcome in neonates was compared with that in older children. In the neonatal group, 80% presented with seizures associated with an acute systemic illness or dehydration, and death or severe residual disability was the final outcome in over 50%. In older children, the underlying cause was an local infection or a prothrombotic state, and the prognosis was much better. In both groups infarction in the Galenic system was more likely to be followed by a lasting neurological deficit than was superficial venous infarction. Shevell *et al.* (1989) give a more optimistic prognosis in neonatal dural sinus thrombosis; 11 out of 12 infants presenting with seizures and with no evidence of birth asphyxia developed normally and had no subsequent seizures. The authors propose that sinus thrombosis is an important and under-recognized cause of seizures in the first 2 weeks of life in term infants.

5

Investigations

COMPUTED TOMOGRAPHY SCAN

Computed tomography (CT) scan with and without contrast injection is usually the first neuroimaging examination carried out, particularly on an emergency basis, in patients with headache, focal deficits or seizures. CT scan is an extremely useful tool to rule out the many conditions that cerebral venous thrombosis (CVT) can mimic. It is also crucial in septic CVT to detect sinus disease, bony abnormalities or changes in the mastoid region. It can also detect other lesions such as meningiomas or abscesses, which can themselves be causes of CVT. Besides ruling out other conditions and sometimes detecting the cause of CVT, CT scan is also useful in showing changes suggestive and occasionally typical of CVT. These changes have been described in detail in numerous reports (Buonanno *et al.*, 1978, 1979, 1982; Kingsley *et al.*, 1978; Brismar, 1980; Ford and Sarwar, 1981; Patronas *et al.*, 1981; Rao *et al.*, 1981; Brant-Zawadzki *et al.*, 1982; Segall *et al.*, 1982; Chiras *et al.*, 1985; Goldberg *et al.*, 1986; Shinohara *et al.*, 1986; Anderson *et al.*, 1987; Virapongse *et al.*, 1987) and are now well established. They can be divided into direct and indirect signs (Table 5.1).

DIRECT SIGNS OF CEREBRAL VENOUS THROMBOSIS

Three abnormalities are considered to be direct signs of CVT: the cord sign; the dense triangle; and the delta or empty triangle sign.

The cord sign

This is visible on unenhanced CT scans and represents the spontaneous visualization of a serpiginous high-density thrombus in a cerebral cortical vein (Buonanno *et al.*, 1978; Ford and Sarwar, 1981; Rao *et al.*, 1981) (Figure 5.1). It is considered as a pathognomonic sign of recent cortical vein thrombosis but it is exceedingly rare: it was present in 2 of 31 cases in Rao's review (1981) and in only 1 of 116 cases in our series. A similar spontaneous increased density can

Table 5.1 CT abnormalities in patients with CVT

CT signs	Virapongse *et al.* (1987)* ($n = 76$)	Ameri and Bousser (1992)† ($n = 91$)	Cantu and Barinagarrementeria (1993)† ($n = 95$)	Daif *et al.* (1995)† ($n = 40$)
Normal	4 (5.3%)	24 (26%)	9 (9.5%)	17 (42%)
Cord sign or dense triangle	5 (6.6%)	0	NI	0
Empty delta	32 (42%)	19 (21%)	32 (34%)	12 (30%)
Falx or tentorium enhancement	5 (6.6%)	17 (19%)	NI	NI
Small ventricles	15 (20%)	47 (52%)	NI	NI
Focal hypodensity	9 (12%)	30 (33%)	23 (24%)	9 (22%)
Focal hyperdensity (haemorrhage)	17 (22%)	18 (20%)	56 (59%)	5 (12.5%)

* Series from literature (from 24 published articles).
† Personal series.
NI, not indicated.

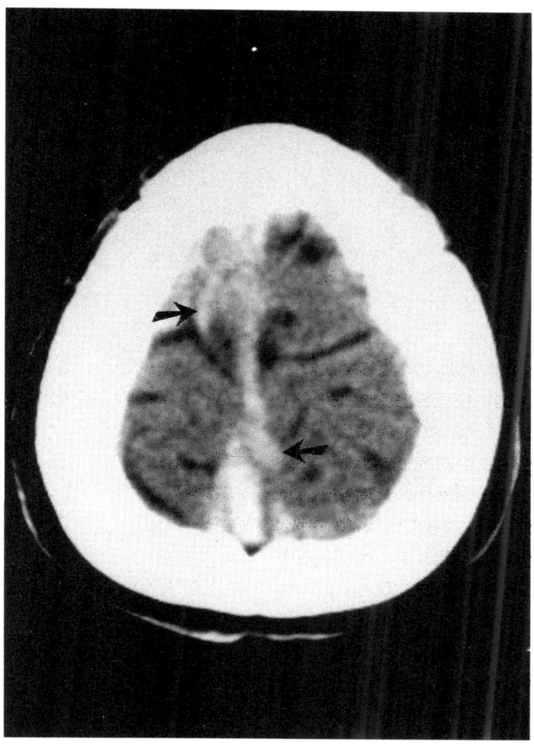

Figure 5.1 An unenhanced CT scan: arrows indicate the 'cord sign' and dense triangle in a SSS thrombosis with thrombosis of adjacent veins. (By courtesy of Professor J. L. Mas, Saint-Anne Hospital, Paris.)

also be seen in lateral sinuses, and in internal cerebral veins and vein of Galen indicating thrombosis of the deep venous system (Ur Rahman and Al-Tahan, 1993) (see Figures 5.17 and 5.18).

The dense triangle sign

This also is visible on unenhanced CT scans and indicates the presence of fresh thrombus in the posterior part of the superior sagittal sinus (SSS) (Patronas *et al.*, 1981; Buonanno *et al.*, 1982) (Figure 5.2). It is thus a very early sign, again

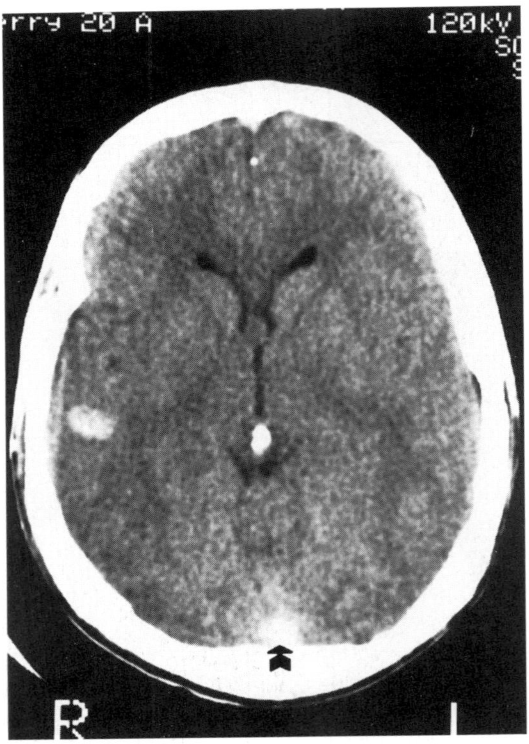

Figure 5.2 An unenhanced CT scan, showing the 'dense triangle' sign in SSS thrombosis (arrow). There is also a small cortical haemorrhage.

extremely rare, present in less than 1 out of 50 cases. Mainly seen in SSS thrombosis, it appears as a strongly hyperdense triangle, which is often difficult to differentiate from the normally slightly hyperdense torcular. An abnormal hyperdensity can also be seen in other sinuses, such as lateral and straight sinuses (Figure 5.3), but again this is difficult to assess because these vessels can be spontaneously hyperdense, particularly in normal children (Osborn *et al.*, 1980) or in dehydrated patients.

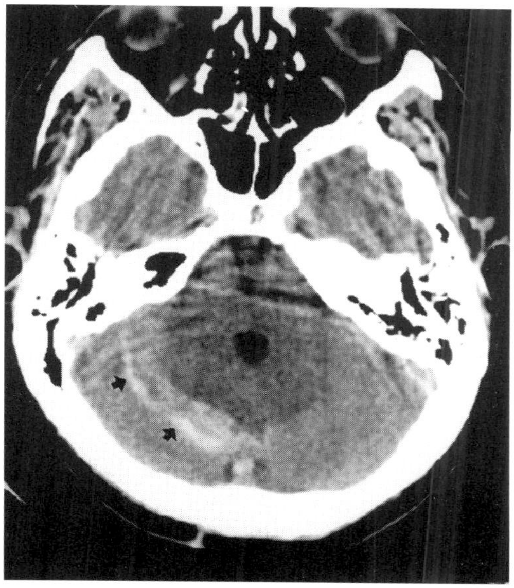

Figure 5.3 An unenhanced CT scan: arrows indicate spontaneous hyperdensity of a thrombosed right lateral sinus.

The empty delta sign (or empty triangle sign)
This was described by Buonanno *et al.* (1978). It appears after contrast injection and is produced by the opacification of the SSS walls contrasting with the low density of the thrombus in the lumen (Figure 5.4). The enhancement of the walls of the sinus is due to the development of collateral venous channels and to the hyperaemia of the dura mater. The empty delta sign is by far the best and most frequent direct sign of CVT, and is present in approximately 35% of published cases (Rao *et al.*, 1981; Buonanno *et al.*, 1982; Anderson *et al.*, 1987; Virapongse *et al.*, 1987). However, its frequency is highly variable according to the site of thrombosis, the timing of the CT scan and the technical parameters employed in this investigation. It was thus present in 72% in Rao's series (1981) of 11 cases but it is found only in 15–20% of CT scans performed routinely to rule out other conditions in patients having symptoms compatible with CVT (Bousser *et al.*, 1985; Chiras *et al.*, 1985). It is absent when thrombosis does not affect the posterior third of SSS or when the CT scan is performed early (in the first 5 days after the onset of symptoms) or late (after 2 months) (Shinohara *et al.*, 1986). Furthermore, although very suggestive of CVT, it is not pathognomonic because the early division of the SSS can be responsible for a false delta sign (Osborn *et al.*, 1980). Despite these restrictions, the delta sign remains the best CT sign of SSS thrombosis. Thus, when there is a clinical suspicion of CVT, this sign must be specifically looked for, which may require some technical refinements, such as orthogonal

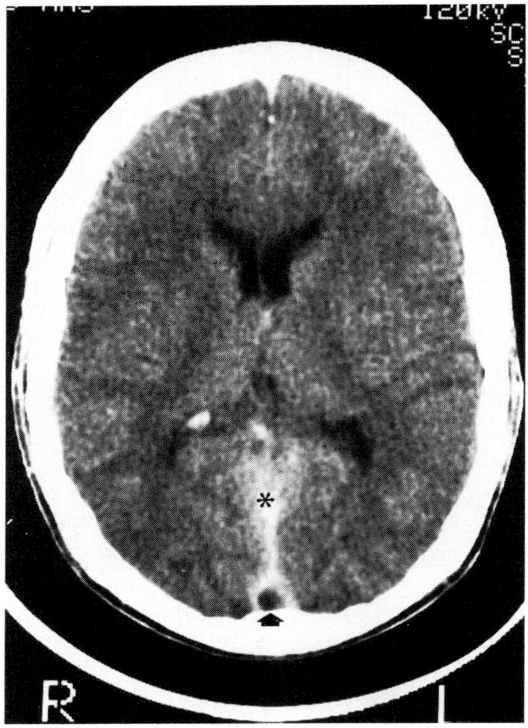

Figure 5.4 A post-contrast CT scan showing the 'empty delta' sign in SSS thrombosis (arrow) with intense tentorial enhancement (asterisk).

sectioning, appropriate window and level settings, and multiplanar reformations (Ford and Sarwar, 1981; Rao *et al.*, 1981; Segall *et al.*, 1982; Goldberg *et al.*, 1986).

INDIRECT SIGNS OF CEREBRAL VENOUS THROMBOSIS

Indirect and non-specific abnormalities are more frequent than direct signs.

Intense contrast enhancement of the falx and tentorium

This is present in some 20% of cases (Buonanno *et al.*, 1978, 1982; Rao *et al.*, 1981; Chiras *et al.*, 1985) (Figure 5.4). It is easily recognized in the tentorium but can be difficult to assess in the falx, particularly in aged patients. It indicates venous stasis or hyperaemia of the dura mater. Tentorial enhancement is usually thought to suggest straight sinus thrombosis (Rao *et al.*, 1981) but it is not rare in thrombosis involving the posterior half of SSS (Bousser *et al.*, 1985; Chiras *et al.*, 1985).

Dilated transcerebral medullary veins

Another less well recognized sign is the visualization on post-contrast CT of dilated transcerebral medullary veins appearing as numerous enhancing vascular structures within the deep white matter and along the grey–white matter junction (Anderson *et al.*, 1987). This sign indicates a major venous stasis usually in relation with an extensive SSS thrombosis. It is, however, a rare sign present in 5% in a recent Mexican series (Barinagarrementeria *et al.*, 1992).

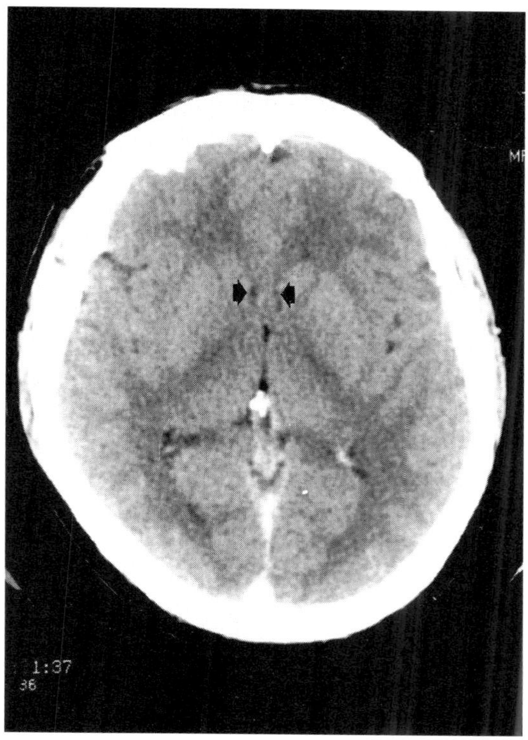

Figure 5.5 Small ventricles in SSS thrombosis (arrows).

Small ventricles

A common finding is the presence of small ventricles resulting from cerebral swelling (Figure 5.5) (Buonanno *et al.*, 1978; Kingsley *et al.*, 1978; Rao *et al.*, 1981; Bousser *et al.*, 1985; Chiras *et al.*, 1985). It is reported in 20–50% of cases, usually in association with other abnormalities. It can, however, be the only sign, in up to 20% of cases. When isolated, it is not a useful sign because of the difficulty in its assessment and its lack of specificity. It is frequently impossible to differentiate small from normal ventricles, particularly in the young. In some

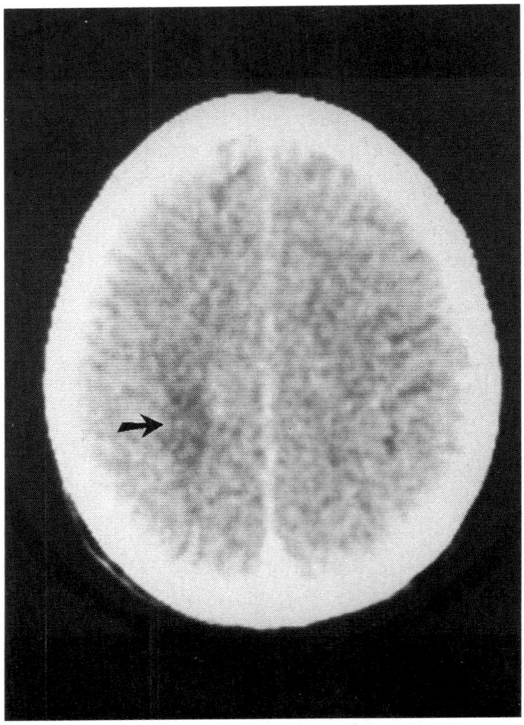

Figure 5.6 A post-contrast CT scan showing a small hypodensity without contrast enhancement in a cortical vein thrombosis (arrow).

cases it is only in retrospect that the initial presence of small ventricles can be confirmed by a subsequent increase in size (Kingsley *et al.*, 1978). Even when definitely present, the finding of small ventricles is in no way specific. It can result from brain swelling from any cause, such as space occupying lesions, brain abscess, encephalitis or benign intracranial hypertension, this last entity being one of the most important differential diagnosis of CVT. Whereas in the majority of CVT cases, ventricles are either small or normal, they can occasionally be enlarged, particularly in cerebellar vein thrombosis (Stevens and Ammerman, 1959; Bousser *et al.*, 1985; Rousseaux *et al.*, 1988).

White matter hypodensity without contrast enhancement

This is suggestive of cerebral oedema and is present in up to 75% of cases (Ford and Sarwar, 1981). It is easier to interpret in adults than in children; it is particularly difficult to assess in the neonate because a similar aspect can be produced by non-myelinated white matter (Ford and Sarwar, 1981). Low-density lesions can be bilateral and diffuse or localized (Figure 5.6). They are sometimes associated with a mass effect with ventricle displacement and sulci

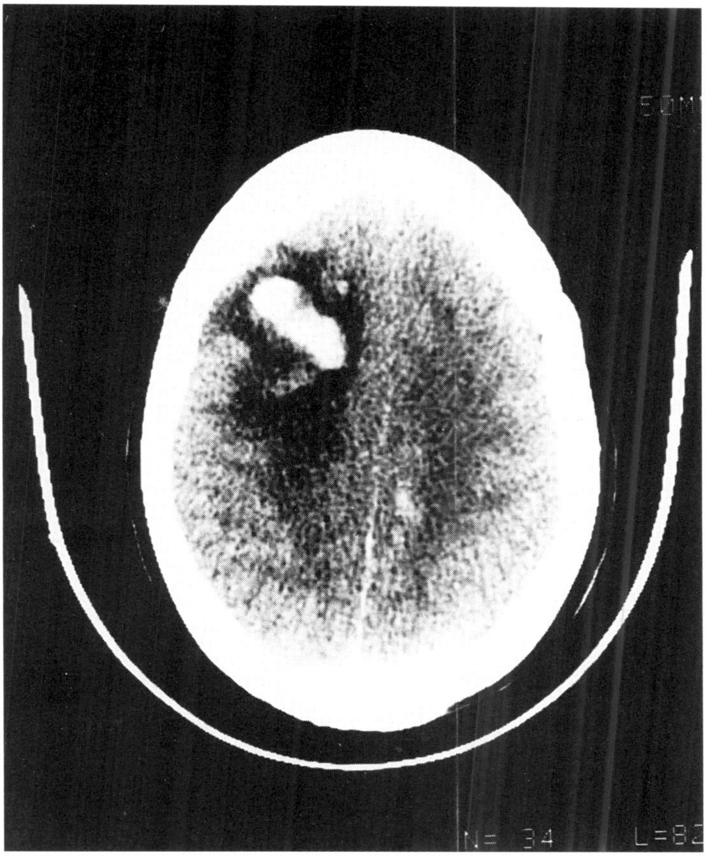

Figure 5.7 Bilateral haemorrhages: small on the left side and large on the right with massive oedema in SSS thrombosis.

disappearance. Brain oedema can be the only parenchymal consequence of CVT but is more often associated with abnormalities suggestive of a venous infarct.

Venous infarcts

These may produce various changes on CT (listed below).

Spontaneously hyperdense haemorrhagic infarcts. These are the most frequent, being present in 10–50% of cases (Rao *et al.*, 1981; Buonanno *et al.*, 1982; Bousser *et al.*, 1985; Chiras *et al.*, 1985; Hanigan *et al.*, 1986). Their size is extremely variable. In the majority of cases, haemorrhages are small, surrounded either by a normal parenchyma or by a hypodensity of variable size (Chiras *et al.*, 1985) (Figure 5.7). Such small haemorrhages are usually multiple (Figure 5.8). Large haemorrhages have also been reported (Estanol

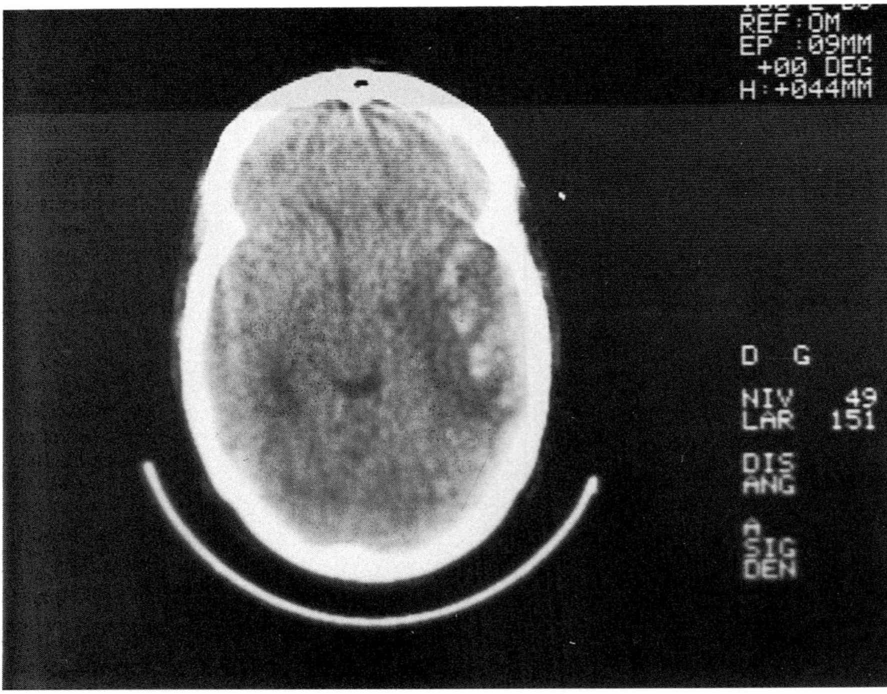

Figure 5.8 Multiple small haemorrhages in a large hypodensity. This is a typical aspect of a haemorrhagic infarct. Important mass effect is shown with a collapsed left ventricle. SSS and cortical veins thrombosis. Reproduced with permission from Bousser *et al.* (1985) Cerebral venous thrombosis: A review of 38 cases. *Stroke* **16**: 199–213. Copyright (1985) American Heart Association.

et al., 1979; Chiras *et al.*, 1985), which may be difficult to differentiate from spontaneous intracerebral haematomas: their subcortical and often scattered location, and their irregular margins are in favour of a venous haemorrhagic infarct. In rare instances, such haemorrhage can be associated with subarachnoid haemorrhage or subdural haematoma (Chiras *et al.*, 1985), which can even be the only CT sign of CVT.

Non-haemorrhagic venous infarcts. These are almost as frequent as haemorrhagic infarcts, being present in 10–40% of cases. They are protean in appearance. The most frequent pattern is that of a subcortical hypodensity with contrast enhancement and varying degrees of mass effect (Figures 5.9–5.11). The enhancement is mostly gyral or immediately subcortical, but other appearances have been reported such as patchy areas (Figure 5.12) or rounded lesions sometimes mimicking metastases, particularly when multiple (Chiras *et al.*, 1985) (Figure 5.13). In some cases, there is no spontaneous

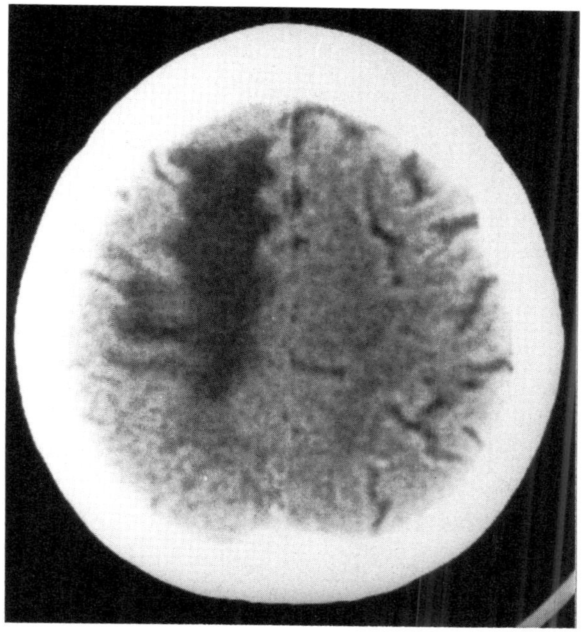

Figure 5.9 Massive subcortical hypodensity in SSS thrombosis.

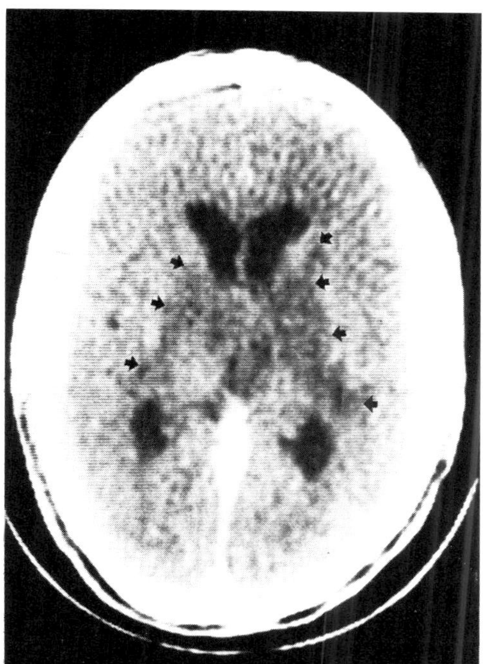

Figure 5.10 Bilateral thalamo-lenticular hypodensity in thrombosis of the deep venous system (indicated by arrows).

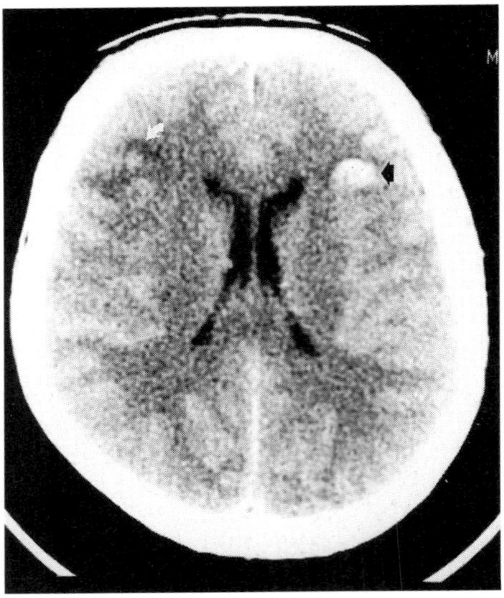

Figure 5.11 A post-contrast CT in SSS thrombosis. A small hypodense area in the right frontal lobe and a nodular enhancement in the left frontal lobe can be seen.

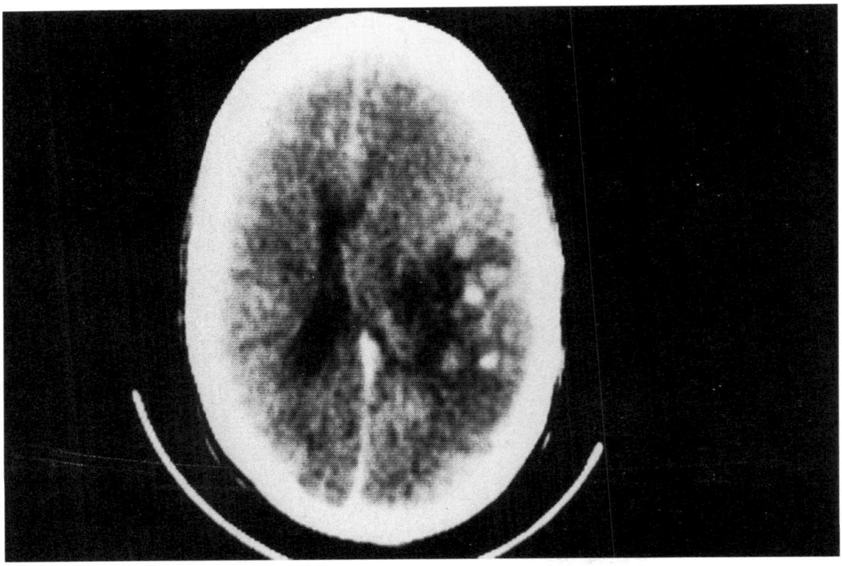

Figure 5.12 A post-contrast CT in SSS and cortical vein thrombosis. Multiple nodular enhancing lesions in an extensive hypodensity with a severe mass effect on the left ventricle can be seen.

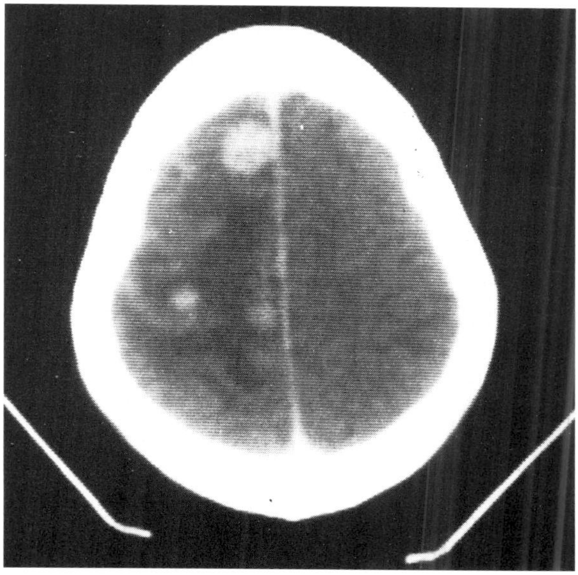

Figure 5.13 A SSS thrombosis. There is a large right subcortical hypodensity with nodular enhancement mimicking metastasis.

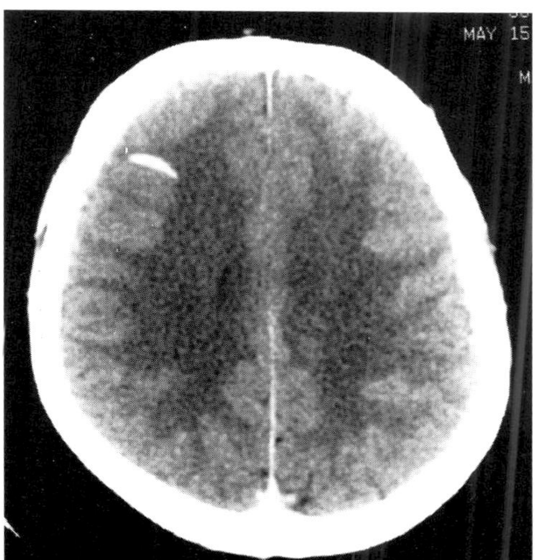

Figure 5.14 Cortical linear enhancement in SSS and cortical vein thrombosis.

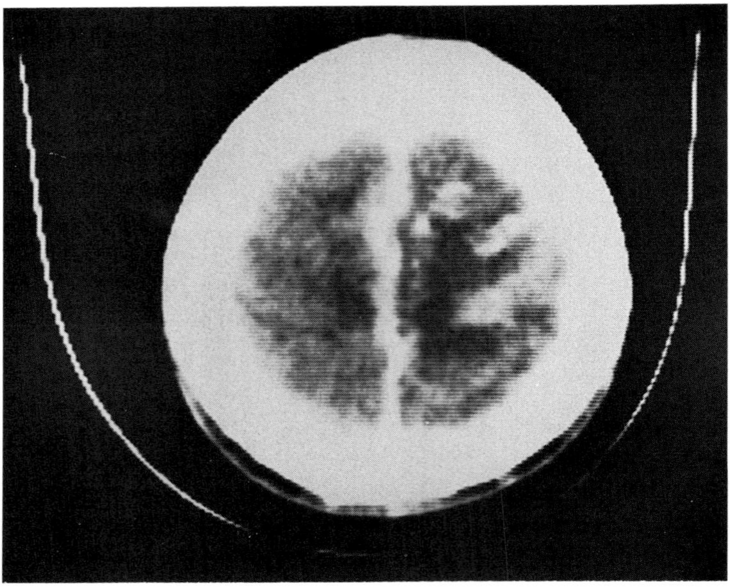

Figure 5.15 A SSS thrombosis with bilateral hypodensity, and intense gyral and falx enhancement. Reproduced with permission from Bousser *et al.* (1985) Cerebral venous thrombosis: A review of 38 cases. *Stroke* **16**: 199–213. Copyright (1985) American Heart Association.

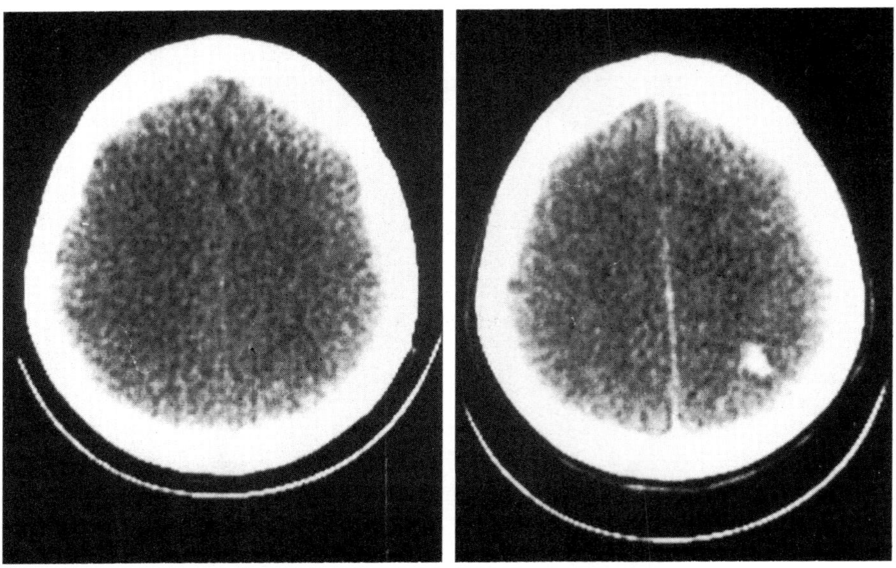

Figure 5.16 No lesion is shown on unenhanced CT scan (left). There is a small area of enhancement in a cortical vein thrombosis (right).

hypodensity and the only anomaly is an isolated contrast enhancement, again highly variable in size and shape: linear (Figure 5.14), gyral (Figure 5.15) or nodular (Figure 5.16).

Haemorrhagic or non-haemorrhagic infarcts. These can be unilateral or bilateral, single or multiple (Bousser *et al.*, 1985; Buonanno *et al.*, 1978, 1982; Rao *et al.*, 1981; Chiras *et al.*, 1985). They are often associated with oedema and with a mass effect, which can occasionally be prominent. They never correspond to the distribution of an arterial territory. They most often complicate SSS thrombosis and are then located superficially, involving both the cortex and the adjacent white matter. In thrombosis of the deep venous system, infarcts are commonly bilateral and less frequently haemorrhagic. They involve all or parts of the corresponding territory, which includes basal ganglia, the surrounding white matter and the upper midbrain (Coquillat and Warter, 1976; Haley *et al.*, 1989; Baumgartner and Landis, 1992; Ur Rahman and Al-Tahan, 1993) (Figures 5.17 and 5.18). Cerebellar venous infarcts can again be either hypodense (with or without contrast enhancement) (Rousseaux *et al.*, 1988) or hyperdense (Eng *et al.*, 1990), and unilateral or bilateral. They are usually associated with compression of the fourth ventricle with secondary hydrocephalus (Eng *et al.*, 1990; Rousseaux, 1988) (Figure 5.19).

CAVERNOUS SINUS THROMBOSIS

This is difficult to diagnose on CT scan, even with intravenous contrast (Clifford–Jones *et al.*, 1982; Goldberg *et al.*, 1986; Deslegte *et al.*, 1988; DiNubile, 1988). Associated signs might be indirectly helpful, such as dilated superior ophthalmic veins or cerebral venous infarcts. The infusion of higher doses of contrast material followed by rapid sequential views of the cavernous sinuses, the use of thin slices (3 mm) complemented by multiplanar reconstruction and direct coronal scanning improve the diagnostic yield (Goldberg *et al.*, 1986; Deslegte *et al.*, 1988). A suggestive appearance is on post-contrast CT that of multiple irregular filling defects with bulging cavernous sinuses and enlarged orbital veins (Chung *et al.*, 1988; Deslegte *et al.*, 1988). The presence of air, seen on coronal sections, has been reported in a case of septic thrombosis (Curnes *et al.*, 1987).

NORMAL CT SCAN

In 10–20% of cases, the CT scan is normal in patients with proven CVT. To these should be added the cases (10–20%) with small ventricles as the only sign. Given the difficulty of interpretation of small ventricles, it can be said that in about 25% of CVT cases, CT scan is normal. The proportion reaches 50% or more in patients presenting with isolated intracranial hypertension but is below 10% in those presenting with focal signs (Rao *et al.*, 1981; Chiras *et al.*, 1985).

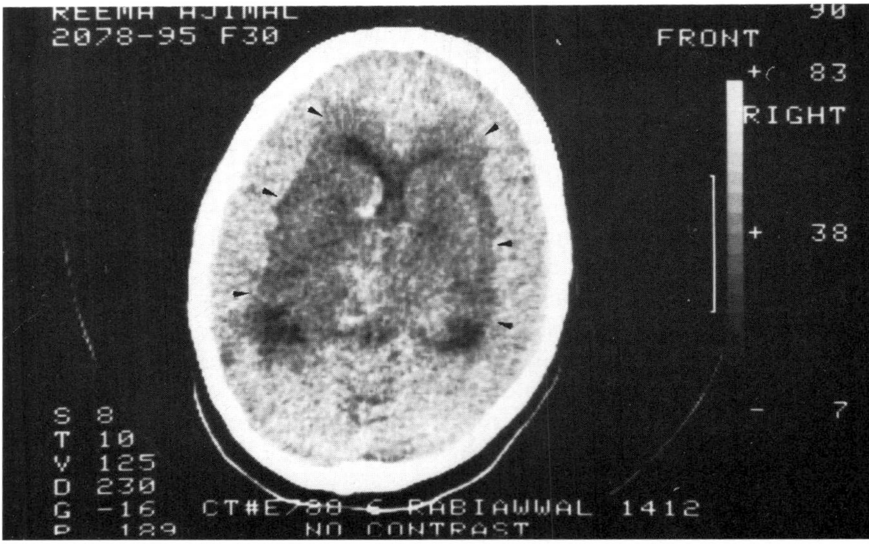

Figure 5.17 A CT scan without contrast: arrows show deep vein thrombosis with extensive hypodensity of deep centrobasilar areas and increased density of the left caudate vein. Reproduced with permission from Ur Rahman and Al-Tahan (1993) Computed tomographic evidence of an extensive thrombosis and infarction of the deep venous system. *Stroke* **24**: 744–746. Copyright (1993) American Heart Association.

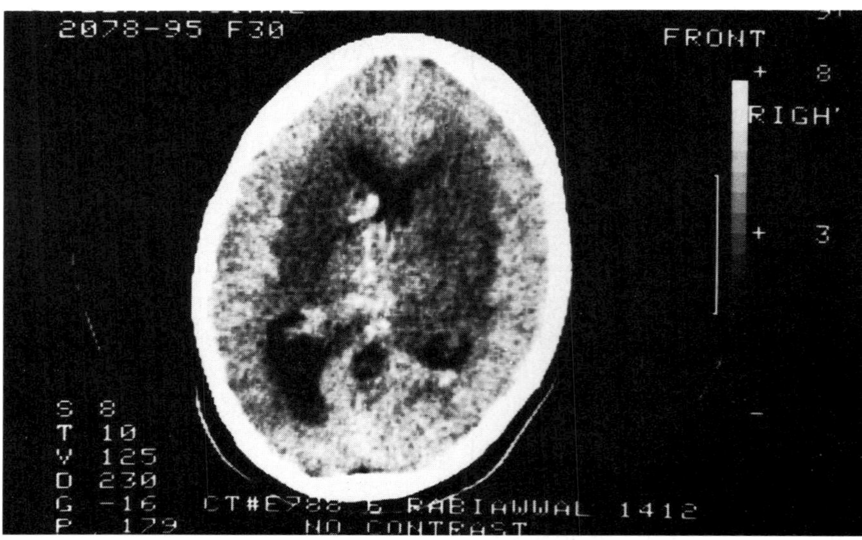

Figure 5.18 A CT scan without contrast (same patient as in Figure 5.17 at a later stage) showing extensive thrombosis of the deep venous system with bilateral infarction of inner basilar structures. Reproduced with permission from Ur Rahman and Al-Tahan (1993) Computed tomographic evidence of an extensive thrombosis and infarction of the deep venous system. *Stroke* **24**: 744–746. Copyright (1993) American Heart Association.

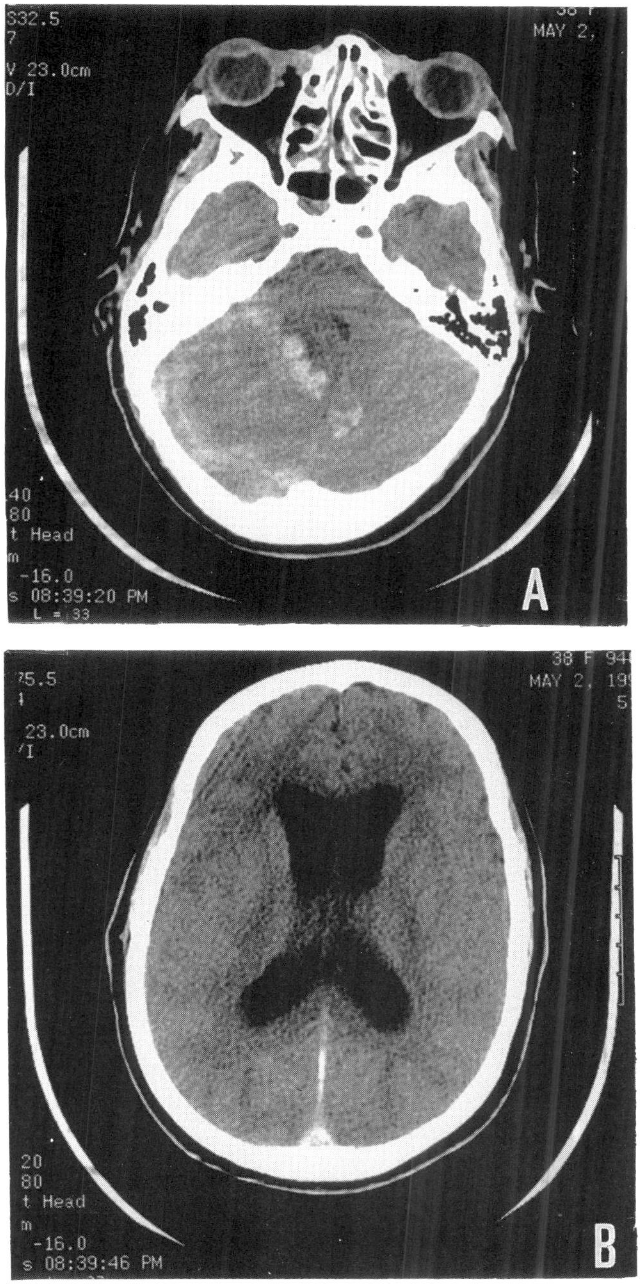

Figure 5.19 A CT scan without contrast showing extensive thrombosis of SSS, right lateral sinus and cerebellar vein with a haemorrhagic cerebellar infarct (A), and hydrocephalus (B).

SUMMARY

The place of CT scan in the diagnostic strategy of CVT differs according to the clinical presentation. When there is a clinical suspicion of CVT, the CT scan has now been supplanted by magnetic resonance imaging (MRI), which should be the initial investigation. However, in many cases, clinical signs are misleading, suggesting other conditions, such as stroke, tumours, abscess or encephalitis, in which CT scan is still often the first investigation, particularly on an emergency basis. Performed first without contrast and, if necessary, with contrast, it usually rules out these conditions easily and frequently reveals abnormalities suggestive of CVT. Nevertheless, since most of these abnormalities are non-specific and may even be absent, MRI or angiographic confirmation should be obtained in all cases lacking CT pathognomonic changes (Bousser *et al.*, 1985; Thron *et al.*, 1986).

ANGIOGRAPHY

INTRA-ARTERIAL ANGIOGRAPHY

Angiography has been the definitive investigation in the diagnosis of CVT for many years and still remains the method of reference for evaluation of new methods. It requires a perfect technique: four-vessel angiography (conventional or digitalized intra-arterial) with visualization of the entire venous phase on at least two projections (frontal and lateral) and, if possible, three oblique views being the best to visualize the entire SSS (Askenasy *et al.*, 1962; Bousser *et al.*, 1985; Krayenbühl, 1954, 1967; Montrieul and Janny, 1962; Vines and Davis, 1971; Yasargil and Damur, 1974). Intravenous digital subtraction angiography is sometimes used in preference to the intra-arterial technique. It is adequate for the detection of sinus occlusion and has the advantage of fewer complications, but it is, at present, not precise enough to assess the veins, the collateral circulation, or a partial filling defect properly (Figure 5.20).

The lack of filling of veins or sinuses
This is the only direct and by far the best angiographic sign of CVT. Easily recognized when it affects the posterior part (Figure 5.21) or the entire SSS (Figure 5.22), both lateral sinuses (LSs) (Figure 5.23) or the straight sinus (Yoshii *et al.*, 1978) (Figure 5.24), it may be more difficult to interpret in other locations, such as the anterior third of the SSS or the left LS, where it can be confused with hypoplasia (Hacker, 1974). To detect occlusion of the anterior part of SSS, it is necessary to have either involvement of another sinus or unequivocal indirect signs of CVT, such as delayed emptying and dilated collateral veins. Another limitation of angiography in SSS thrombosis is the presence of a congenitally bifurcated sinus. This anatomical variant is present in about 2% of subjects (Hosley *et al.*, 1991). If only one of the channels is thrombosed, it may be

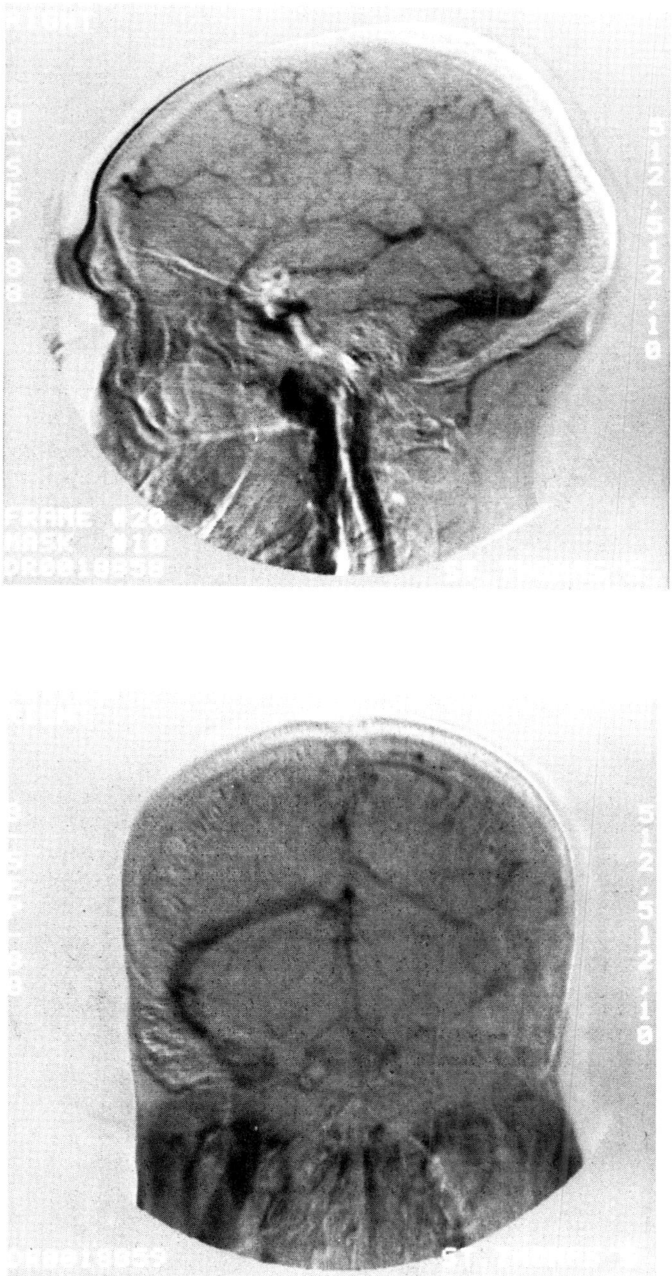

Figure 5.20 Intravenous digital subtraction angiography. There is a lack of filling of the SSS and left transverse sinus.

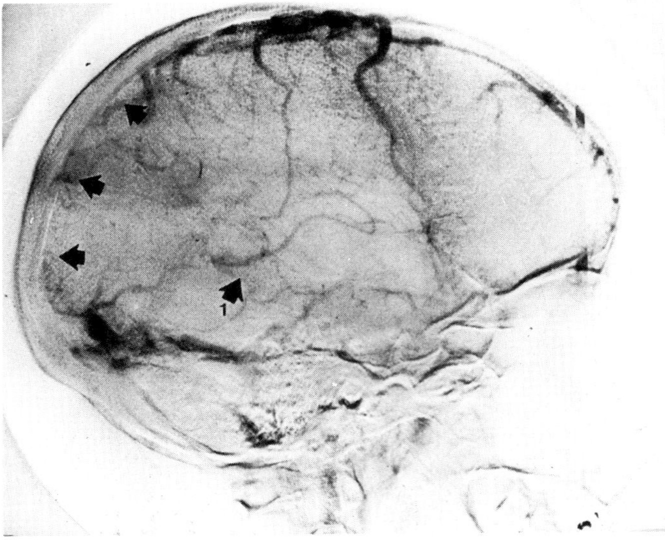

Figure 5.21 Thrombosis of the posterior part of the SSS and of the basal vein of Rosenthal (1) (arrows).

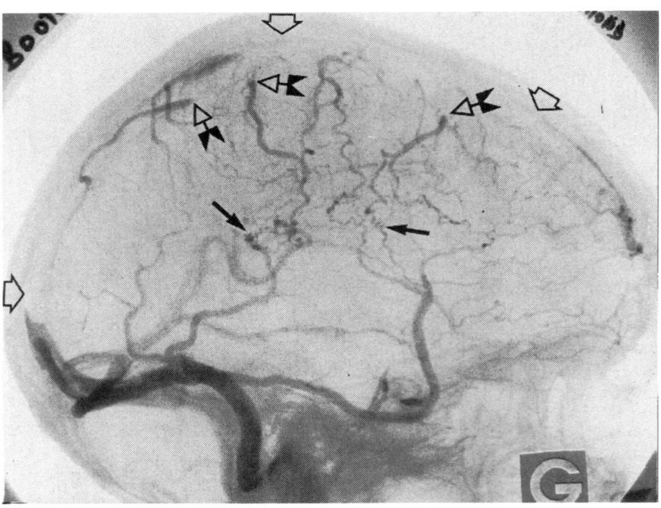

Figure 5.22 Non-injection of the entire SSS (open arrow). The abrupt ending of cortical vein (open arrow with black end) and dilated 'corkscrew' vessels (black arrow) are shown. Thrombosis of the entire SSS and adjacent cortical veins. Reproduced with permission from Bousser *et al.* (1985) Cerebral venous thrombosis. A review of 38 cases. *Stroke* **16**: 199–213. Copyright (1985) American Heart Association.

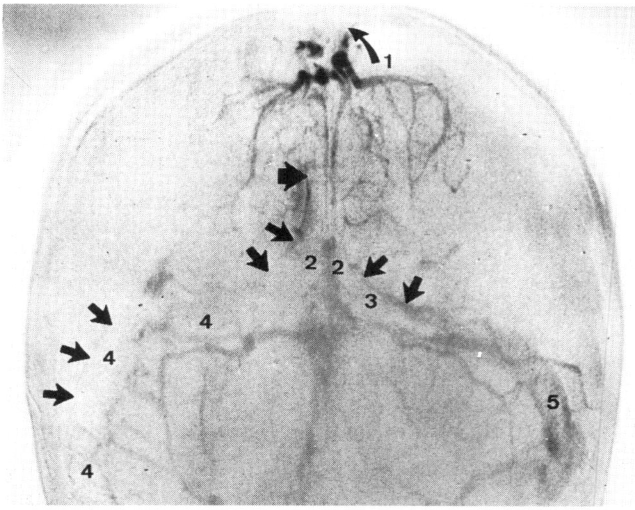

Figure 5.23 Non-injection of the entire SSS (1) and of both LSs (2, 3, 4). Only the sigmoid portion of the left LS is injected (5) (indicated by arrows).

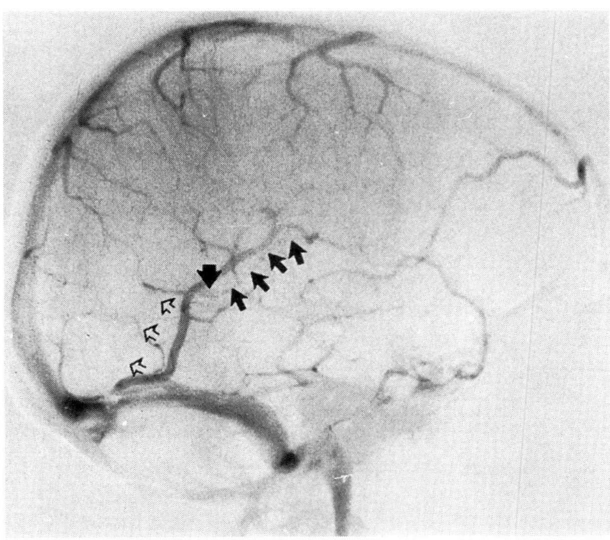

Figure 5.24 Thrombosis of the entire deep venous system internal cerebral vein (thin arrow), vein of Galen (thick arrow), straight sinus (open arrow). Reproduced with permission from Bousser *et al.* (1985), Copyright American Heart Association.

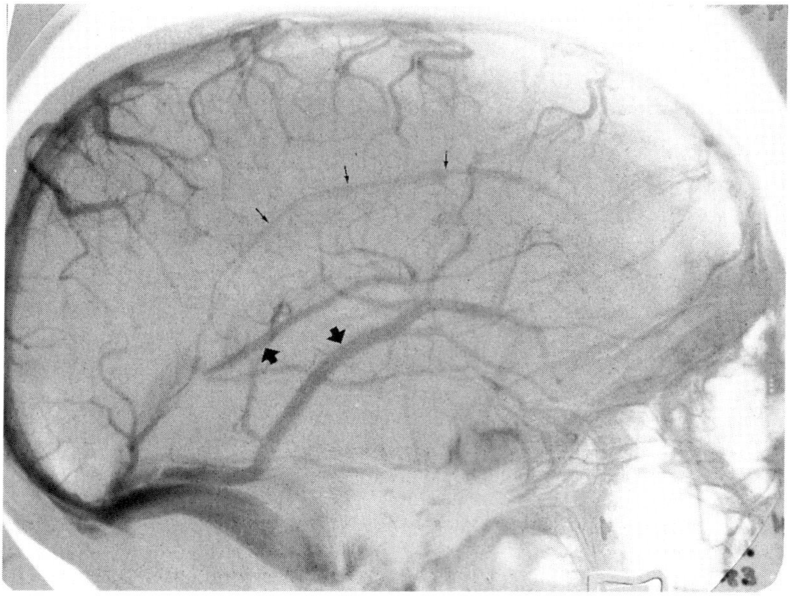

Figure 5.25 Thrombosis of the internal cerebral vein and vein of Galen, showing abnormal visibility of the inferior sagittal sinus (thin arrows), and enlargement of anastomotic cortical veins (thick arrows).

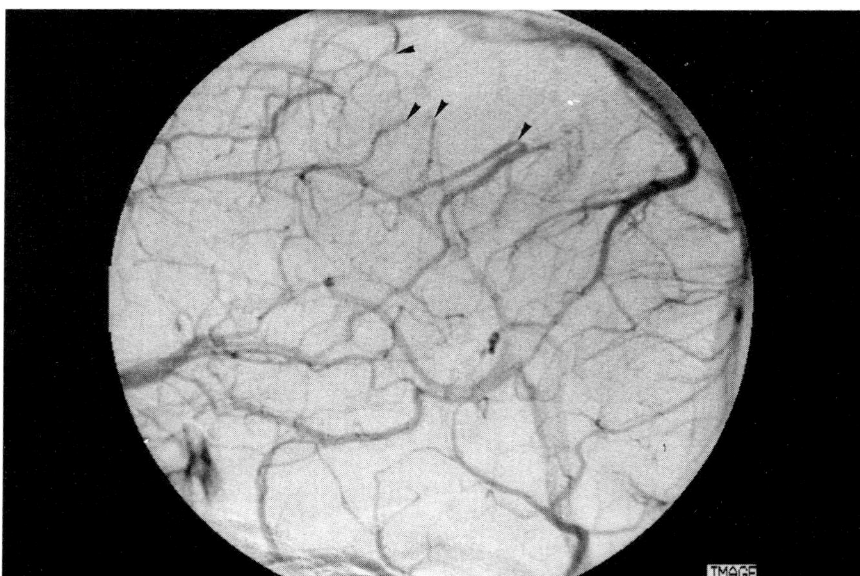

Figure 5.26 Cortical vein thrombosis with veins ending abruptly (arrows).

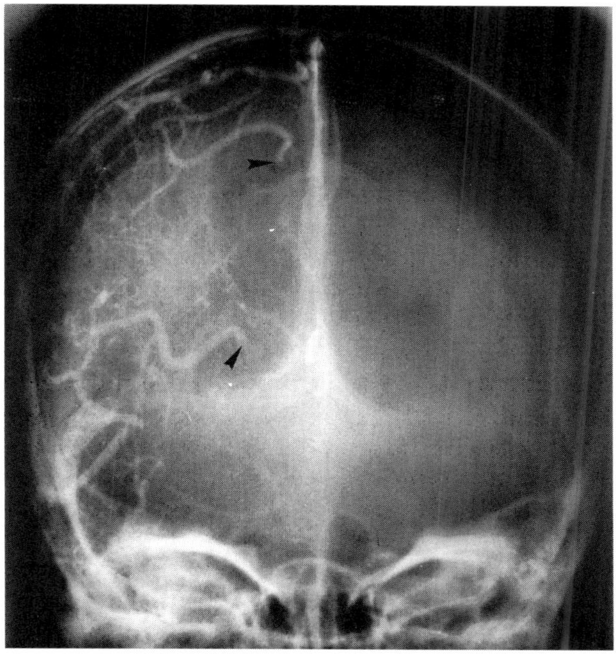

Figure 5.27 Cortical vein and SSS thrombosis with veins ending abruptly (arrows).

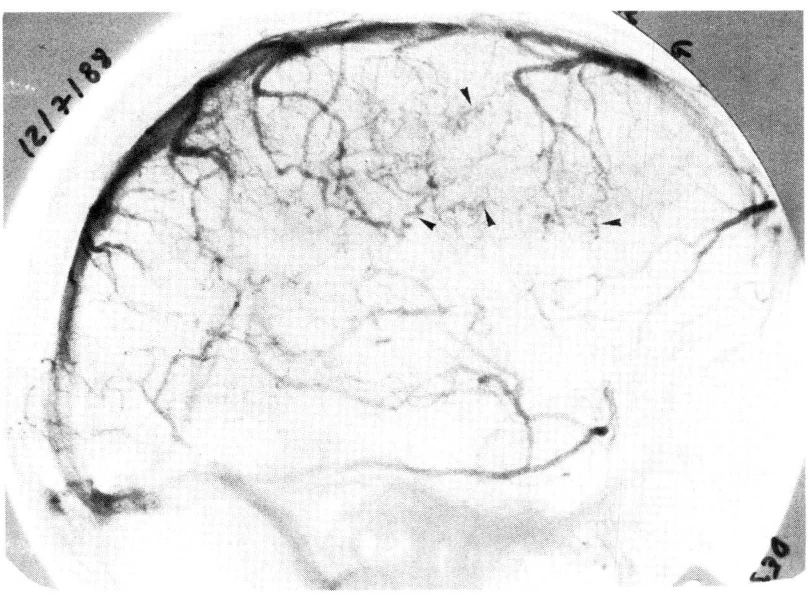

Figure 5.28 Isolated cortical vein thrombosis. One fronto-rolandic vein is missing. There are numerous 'corkscrew' collateral vessels (arrows).

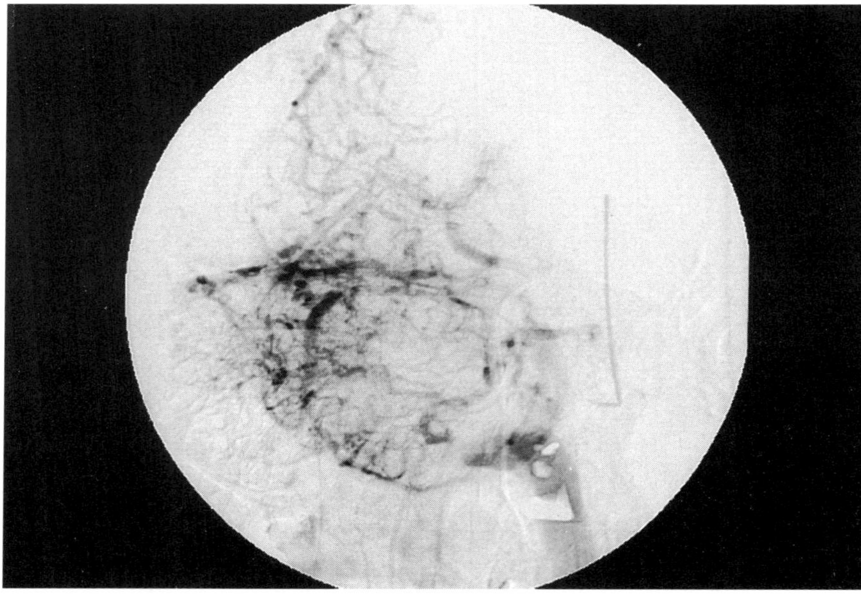

Figure 5.29 An oblique view of the cerebellar veins with dilated 'corkscrew' vessels in a cerebellar vein thrombosis.

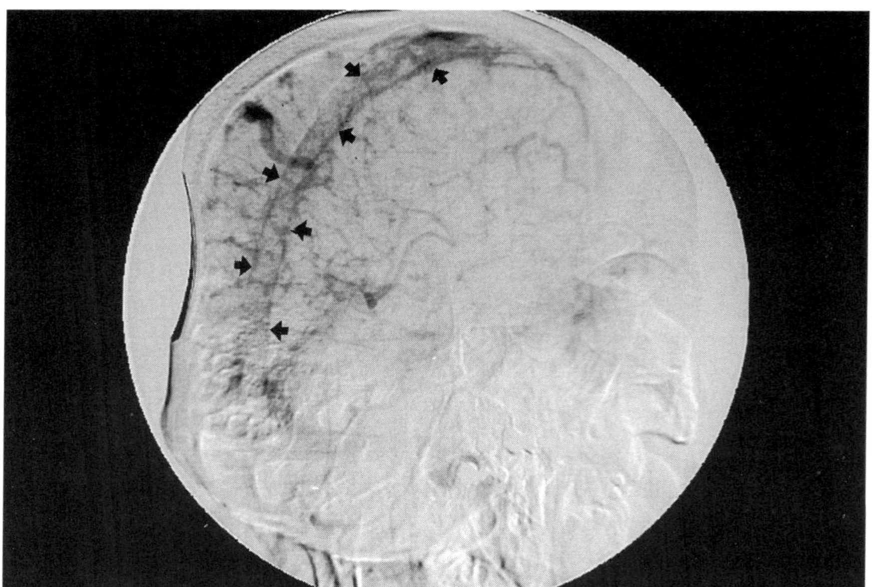

Figure 5.30 An oblique view of SSS, which is filled with an extensive thrombus (indicated by arrows). (By courtesy Dr B. Pertuiset, American Hospital, Paris).

overlooked at angiography but will be revealed at MRI. In LS thrombosis, the important feature is the absence of filling of the whole sinus or of its sigmoid portion in the presence of a normal sinus groove and a normal jugular foramen on plain X-rays of the skull (Buonanno *et al.*, 1979). However, in some cases such signs are lacking and MRI is again required to differentiate between thrombosis and hypoplasia. The non-injection of cerebral veins is easy to recognize in the deep venous system because the basilar and internal cerebral veins are constant, and do not vary in location (Figures 5.21, 5.24 and 5.25). By contrast the absence of a cortical or cerebellar vein is difficult to detect because these veins are variable in number, size and location. When the thrombosis also affects the draining sinus, there is no difficulty, but when it only affects a cortical vein, the appearance can be deceptive. It can only be suspected when a poorly visualized vein ends abruptly (Figures 5.26 and 5.27) ('stop' sign) or when a small avascular area is surrounded by dilated collateral 'corkscrew' veins (Gabrielsen *et al.*, 1981) (Figures 5.28 and 5.29).

In some cases, the thrombosis does not lead to complete occlusion and there is a partial filling of the affected vessel, with rounded filling defects suggestive of intraluminal thrombosi. The diagnosis may then be difficult, particularly in SSS thrombosis, if oblique views are not performed (Figure 5.30).

Delayed emptying and collateral venous pathways

Other angiographic findings include delayed emptying and collateral venous pathways. Delayed emptying is found in 50% of cases (Krayenbühl, 1954; Montrieul and Janny, 1962; Bousser *et al.*, 1985), and explains why in conventional angiography, the venous phase was frequently not visualized and CVT was overlooked. Films taken up to 12 seconds after the injection of contrast were needed (Krayenbühl, 1954). The development of collateral venous pathways is also found in approximately half the cases and almost invariably indicates SSS thrombosis. Three varieties of collateral pathways have been reported according to the site, extent and duration of CVT (Krayenbühl, 1954; Montrieul and Janny, 1962; Greitz and Link, 1966; Kalbag and Woolf, 1967; Vines and Davis, 1971; Yasargil and Damur, 1974; Bousser *et al.*, 1985). Cortical collateral veins are by far the most frequent. They appear as dilated and tortuous veins, with a 'corkscrew' appearance, which often run horizontally between cortical veins or between fronto-parietal veins and vein of Labbé (Figures 5.22, 5.28 and 5.29). These corkscrew vessels are an excellent indirect sign of cortical vein occlusion. Transcerebral anastomosis are less frequent. They occur in extensive thrombosis either of the SSS or of the deep venous system, and can appear either as very fine linear vessels or as large tortuous channels. Collateral veins can also be visualized in the walls of the sagittal sinus. They are represented as thin lines of contrast material adjacent to the occluded lumen of the sinus (Figure 5.31). In extensive and permanent occlusion of SSS and lateral sinus, collateral channels may extend transdurally to anastomose with scalp veins (Greitz and Link, 1966; Kalbag and Woolf, 1967; Vines and Davis, 1971) (Figure 5.32).

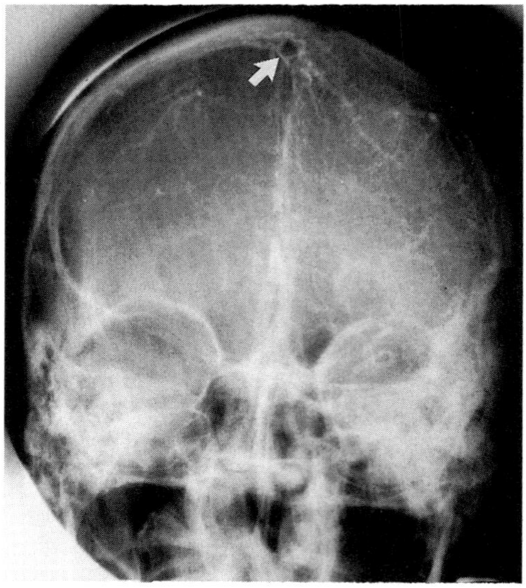

Figure 5.31 SSS thrombosis (indicated by arrows). Collateral circulation in the sinus walls contrasting with the non-injection of the occluded sinus. This is the angiographic equivalent of the empty delta sign.

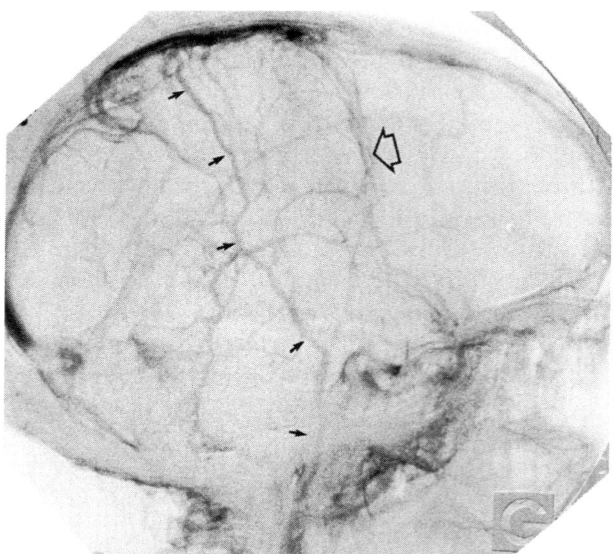

Figure 5.32 Longstanding SSS thrombosis with transdural anastomosis (indicated by arrows). Reproduced with permission from Bousser *et al.* (1985) Cerebral venous thrombosis. A review of 38 cases. *Stroke* **16**: 199–213. Copyright (1985) American Heart Association.

MAGNETIC RESONANCE ANGIOGRAPHY

Magnetic resonance angiography (MRA), combined with MRI now tends to replace intra-arterial angiography for the diagnosis of CVT. There are several methods of visualizing the intracranial veins, including two-dimensional time of flight (2D TOF), three-dimensional (3D) TOF and phase-contrast techniques (Mattle *et al.*, 1990; Rippe *et al.*, 1990; Padayachee *et al.*, 1991; Anderson *et al.*, 1993; Chelly *et al.*, 1994). Each technique has been used effectively for the diagnosis of CVT, although the 2D TOF and phase-contrast techniques have some advantages over the 3D TOF technique (Johnson and Fram, 1992; Anderson *et al.*, 1993).

The most commonly used method is the 2D TOF with 1.5–2 mm thick slices in the coronal and axial planes (Chelly *et al.*, 1994). A presaturation pulse is placed inferiorly to reduce the signal from arterial structures (Mattle *et al.*, 1991). In the coronal plane, there is usually a loss of signal intensity within the torcular Herophili, which can be overcome by rotating the scan plane into a slightly tilted oblique sagittal projection (Anderson *et al.*, 1993). In the axial acquisition, there is also frequently a loss of signal in the mid-portion of the SSS and occasionally within the internal cerebral veins (Anderson *et al.*, 1993).

Another very effective method to image dural sinuses is phase-contrast (PC) angiography, which can be made sensitive to venous flow rates by selecting a velocity encoding of 20 cm s^{-1} (Rippe *et al.*, 1990; Anderson *et al.*, 1993). A sagittal PC slab angiogram is first acquired to study SSS and the deep venous system. A second PC slab angiogram is performed in the axial plane to study lateral sinuses and jugular veins. This technique has the advantage of being sensitive to flow in all directions, of visualizing in plane the flow due to subtraction of background tissue, and of displaying only moving spin (Tsuruda *et al.*, 1991; Anderson *et al.*, 1993). 3D TOF angiography has also been successfully used to diagnose sinus thrombosis (Villringer *et al.*, 1989), but it can give ambiguous results because a subacute intraluminal thrombus containing haemoglobin will appear as an increased signal intensity, thus simulating normal flow (Anderson *et al.*, 1993). Refinements of these three techniques have been proposed to quantify the flow (Mattle *et al.*, 1990, 1991) to determine its direction (Anderson *et al.*, 1993), and to increase the contrast between moving blood and stationary tissue (Padayachee *et al.*, 1991).

The typical appearance of sinus thrombosis on MRA is, as with intra-arterial angiography, the absence of flow, which indicates a complete thrombosis (Figures 5.33–5.35). Partial thrombosis may be more problematic because flow is still present but irregular. Intravenous contrast material might then be useful because it increases the intraluminal signal intensity for slow flow, facilitating the identification of collateral pathways as well as flow around localized thrombus. However, such cases are rare and, in the vast majority, no contrast is required for the MR diagnosis of CVT.

Some specific limitations of MRA have already been discussed, such as the loss of signal intensity owing to saturation of the in-plane flow, particularly

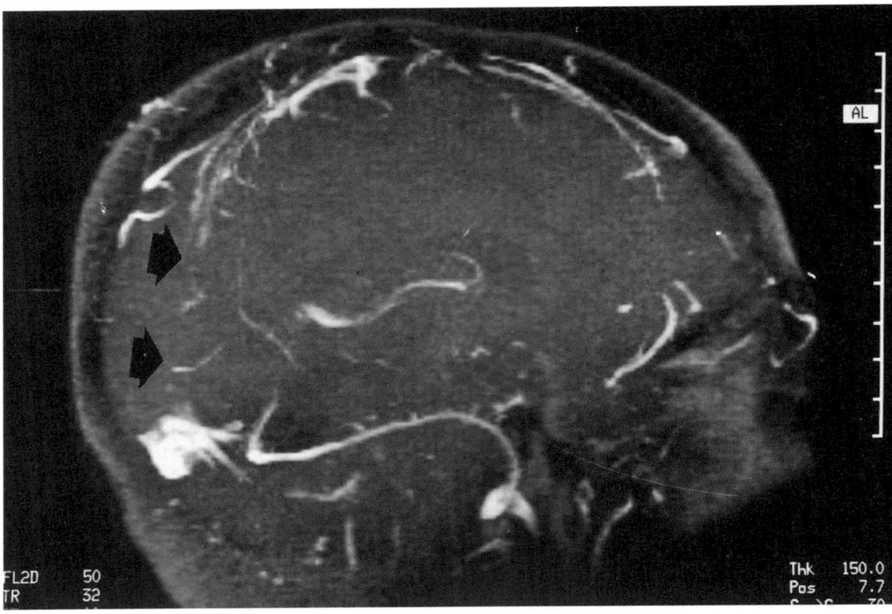

Figure 5.33 Two-dimensional time of flight MRA: thrombosis of the posterior part of the SSS (arrows) and lateral sinus.

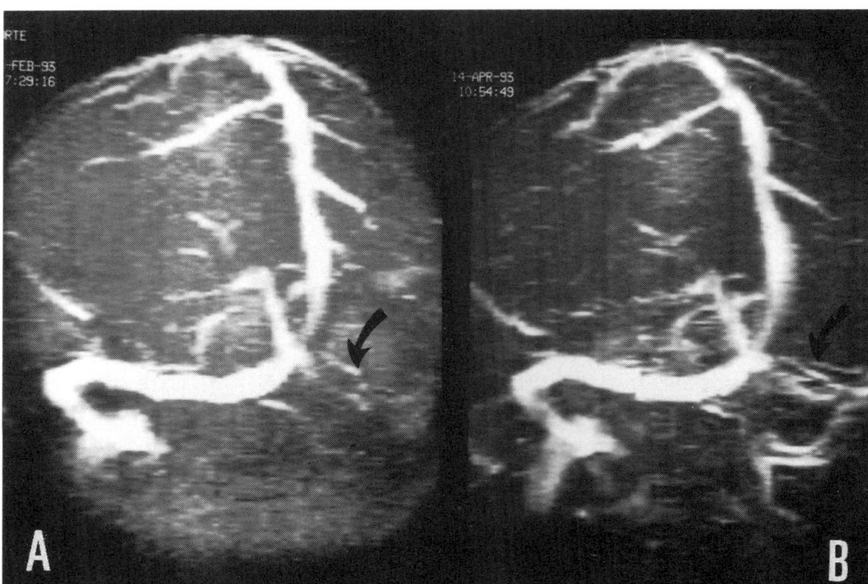

Figure 5.34 Two-dimensional time of flight MRA: arrows indicate thrombosis of the right LS (A) with partial recanalization 2 months later (B).

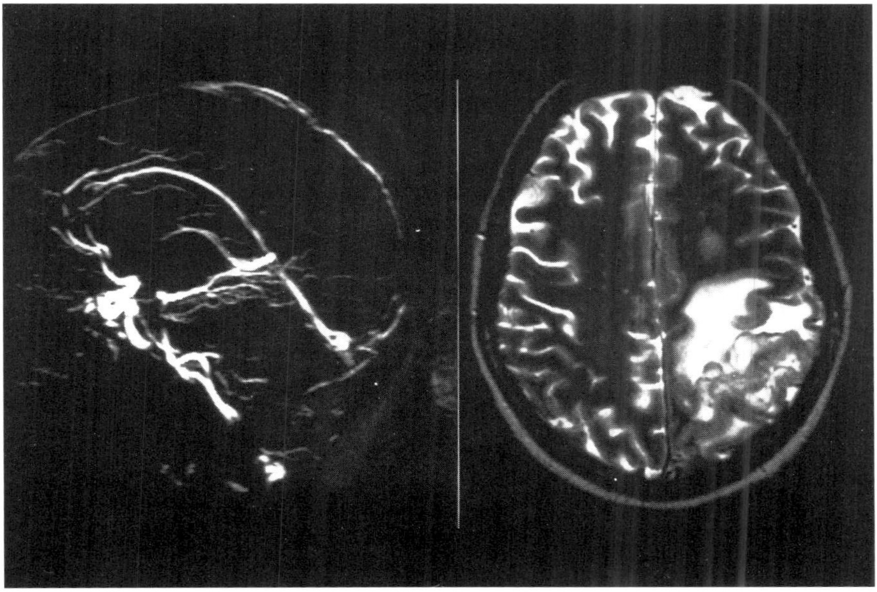

Figure 5.35 Phase-contrast MRA and MRI of partial SSS thrombosis showing poorly visualized SSS at MRA with increased signal of inferior sagittal sinus. A haemorrhagic infarct and oedema are shown on MRI. (By courtesy of Professor Cordoleani, Val de Grâce Hospital, Paris.)

with 2D TOF acquisitions, and the confusion between thrombus and flow, which can occur with the 3D TOF technique. Other limitations are common to all varieties of angiography: the inability to differentiate hypoplasia and thrombosis in the anterior third of the SSS, and, in the LS, the difficulty in identifying cortical vein thrombosis and the very poor diagnostic yield for cavernous sinus thrombosis. In this last condition, the best images are usually obtained by a combination of non-contrast- and contrast-enhanced 2D TOF images (Anderson *et al.*, 1993).

In summary, MRA is tending to replace intra-arterial X-ray angiography to diagnose CVT, but the best diagnostic yield is at present obtained with a combination of MRA and MR imaging.

MAGNETIC RESONANCE IMAGING

MRI offers major advantages for the evaluation of patients suspected of CVT because of its sensitivity to blood flow, its ability to visualize the thrombus itself and its non-invasiveness. It is also more sensitive than CT in detecting parenchymal changes.

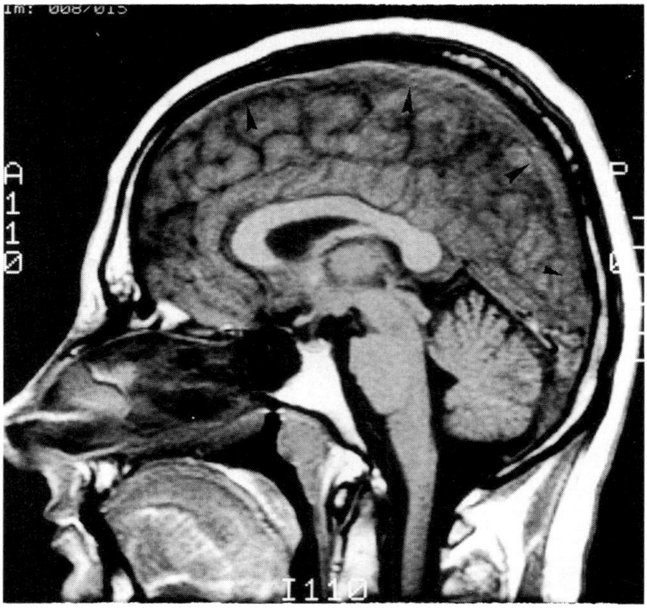

Figure 5.36 T1WI MRI: arrows indicate extensive SSS thrombosis examined at day 3. Isosignal of the entire SSS.

THROMBOSIS IMAGING

Most MRI studies have concentrated on the imaging of sinus thrombosis. A variety of MR findings have been described mainly related to the evolution of thrombosis (Hanigan *et al.*, 1986; Macchi *et al.*, 1986; McMurdo *et al.*, 1986; Savino *et al.*, 1986; Snyder and Sachdev, 1986; Thron *et al.*, 1986; McArdle *et al.*, 1987; Sze *et al.*, 1988; Dormont *et al.*, 1994; Isensee *et al.*, 1994) (Tables 5.2 and 5.3).

At a very early stage, there is an absence of flow void and the occluded vessel appears isointense on T1-weighted imaging (T1WI) and hypointense on T2-weighted imaging (T2WI) (Figure 5.36). Such a pattern is rare since only a minority of CVT patients are examined with MRI in the very first days: it was found in only one case (seen at 24 hours), in a series of 53 patients (Dormont *et al.*, 1994). On the other hand, it was present in all 8 patients examined during the first 5 days in the series of 23 patients reported by Isensee *et al.* (1994). Another early pattern is a high-intensity signal on T1WI and a low-intensity signal on T2WI. This was also seen in one case, studied 4 days after the onset of symptoms, in the same series of 53 cases (Dormont *et al.*, 1994). At a very early stage, the decreased signal of acute thrombosis may be confused with patency. It is one of the very few false negatives of MRI in CVT (Sze *et al.*, 1988). In such cases, it is crucial to perform an MRA, which will demonstrate the absence of flow in the thrombosed sinus. Flow-sensitive gradient echosequences might also be useful in this respect (Daniels *et al.*, 1989).

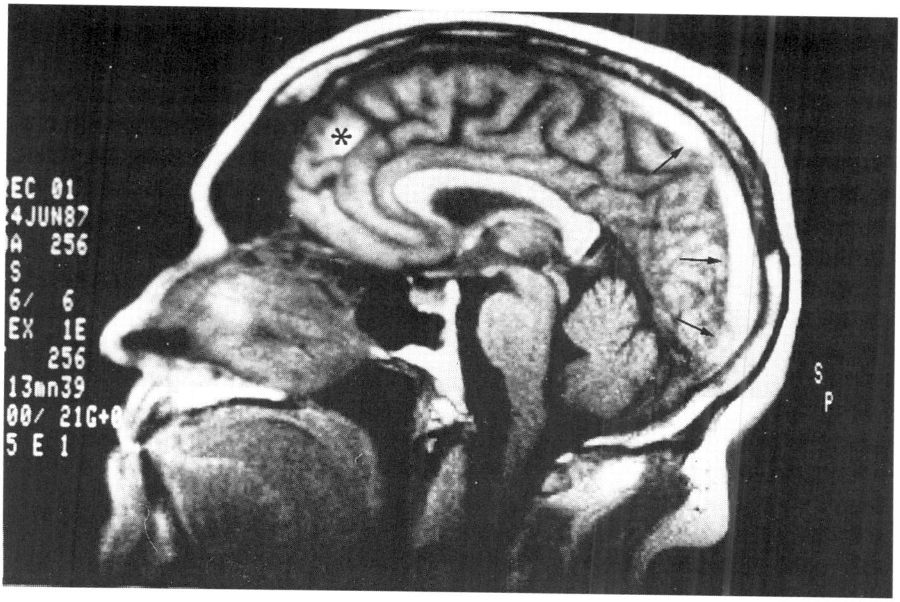

Figure 5.37 T1WI MRI: arrows indicate an increased signal of the thrombosed posterior part of SSS (day 15). There is a small frontal haemorrhage (asterisk).

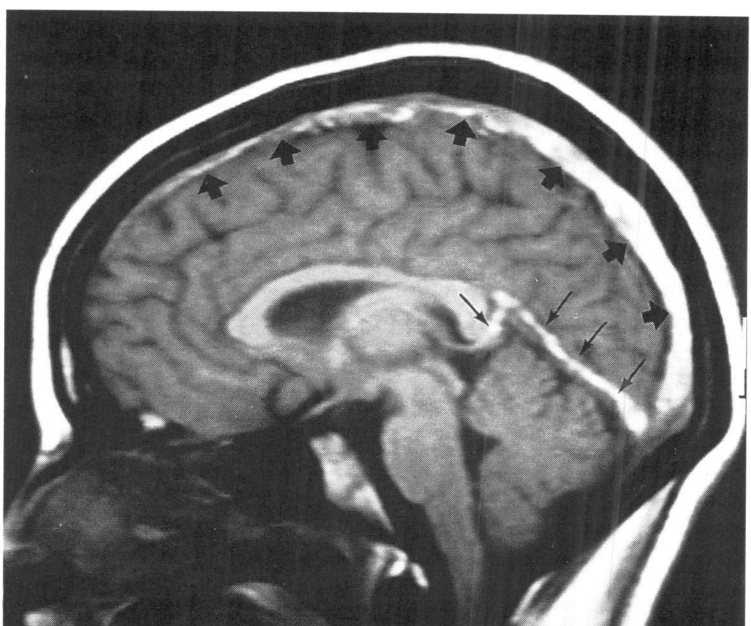

Figure 5.38 T1WI MRI showing increased signal of the entire SSS (thick arrows), vein of Galen and straight sinus (thin arrows) (day 18).

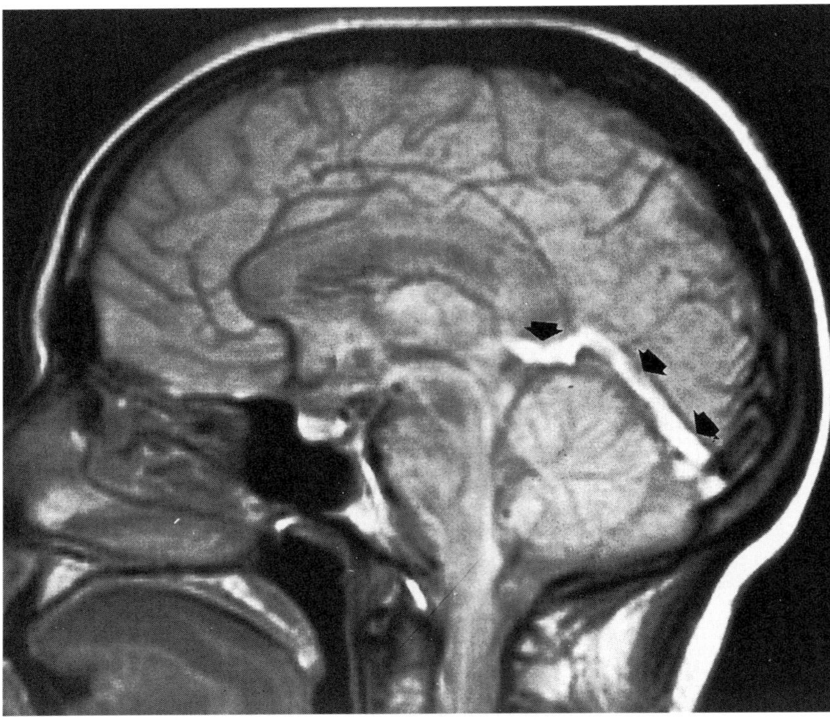

Figure 5.39 T2WI MRI (first echo): arrows indicate thrombosis of the vein of Galen and straight sinus (day 22).

A few days later, the absence of flow void persists but the thrombus becomes hyperintense, initially on T1WI and then on T2WI (Figures 5.37–5.40). In large vessels, these changes start in the periphery and proceed towards the centre. The image is then that of a target consisting of a central isointensity surrounded by a peripheral circumferential hyperintensity. These changes represent the ageing of the thrombus with biochemical conversion of oxyhaemoglobin to methaemoglobin, rather than the extension of thrombosis. This intermediate pattern (increased signal in T1 and T2WI) is the most frequent one. It was found in 12 out of 28 cases in Ameri and Bousser's series (1992) and in 34 out of 53 in Dormont's series (1994). The exact timing of the appearance and disappearance of this pattern is not known, but it is usually found between days 4 or 5, and days 30 to 35 of the onset of symptoms.

After the first month, MRI patterns are variable, since the thrombosed vessel can either remain totally or partially occluded, or recanalize and return to normal (Figures 5.41–5.43). In the majority of cases, during the second month, there is an isosignal on T1WI and an increased signal on T2WI. This pattern was found in 14 of 53 cases in Dormont's series (1994). At that stage, flow-sensitive

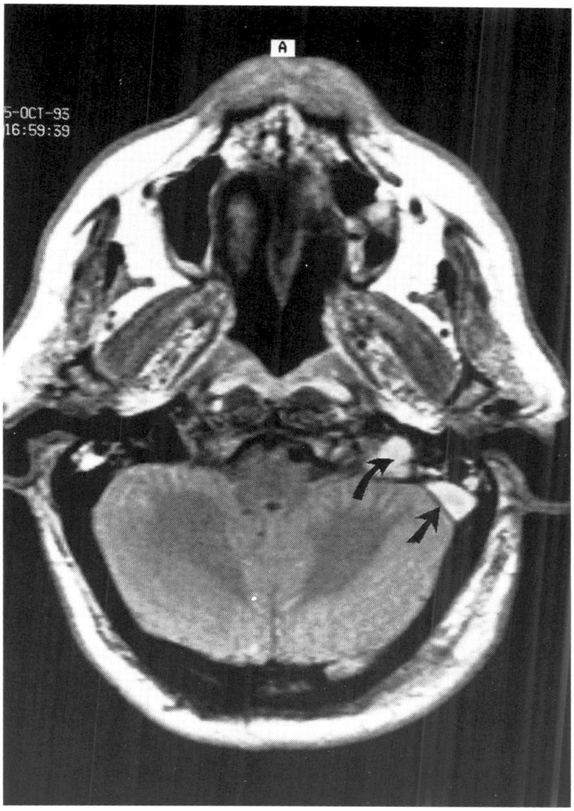

Figure 5.40 T2WI MRI: arrows indicate increased signal of the thrombosed LS and internal jugular vein (day 17).

Table 5.2 MRI patterns of sinus thrombosis according to the type of sequence and the stage of thrombosis

	Normal	Sinus thrombosis		
		Early < day 5	Intermediate (1st month	Late* (> 1 month)
SET1	Variable	Isosignal	High signal	Isosignal
SET2	No signal	Low signal	High signal	High or isosignal
GE	High signal	Isosignal	High signal	Hyper or isosignal

* Abnormalities indicated here are the most frequent ones but in approximately 30% of cases, the signal can be entirely back to normal.
SET1, spin echo T1-weighted images; SET2, spin echo T2-weighted images; GE, flow-sensitive gradient echo sequences.

gradient echosequences are useful to confirm the persistent occlusion, which shows on these sequences as an isosignal (Daniels *et al.*, 1989).

At 6 months, persistent abnormalities are observed in more than two thirds of cases. They are usually more limited in length, involving only part of a sinus. The signal of this chronic thrombus is often heterogeneous but predominantly isointense on T1WI, and hypertense or isointense to brain parenchyma on T2WI (Mas *et al.*, 1992) (Figure 5.44). These abnormalities can persist for years (Dormont *et al.*, 1994) and should not be mistaken for a recurrent acute CVT. By contrast, in a minority of cases [2 out of 21 in one series (Isensee *et al.*, 1994), one third in another (Mas *et al.*, 1992)], sinuses are entirely normal at 6 months, which does not allow a retrospective diagnosis.

Table 5.3 Spin echo MRI patterns in two series of CVT.

	Dormont *et al.* (1994) (n = 53)	Ameri and Bousser (1992) (n = 28)
Iso T1 + low T2	1 (day 1)	0
High T1 + low T2	1 (day 4)	0
High T1 + high T2	34 (m = 20 days)	12 (day 1–30)
Iso T1 + high T2	14 (30–60 days)	6 (> day 30)
Normal T1 + high T2	0	7 (> day 30)
Normal T1 and T2	3	3

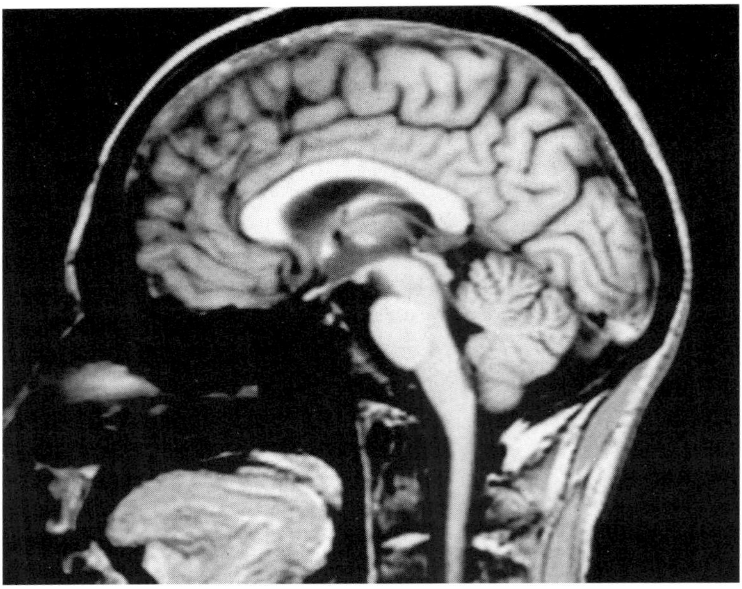

Figure 5.41 T1WI MRI showing SSS thrombosis at 5 weeks. There is a partial recanalization of the posterior part of SSS.

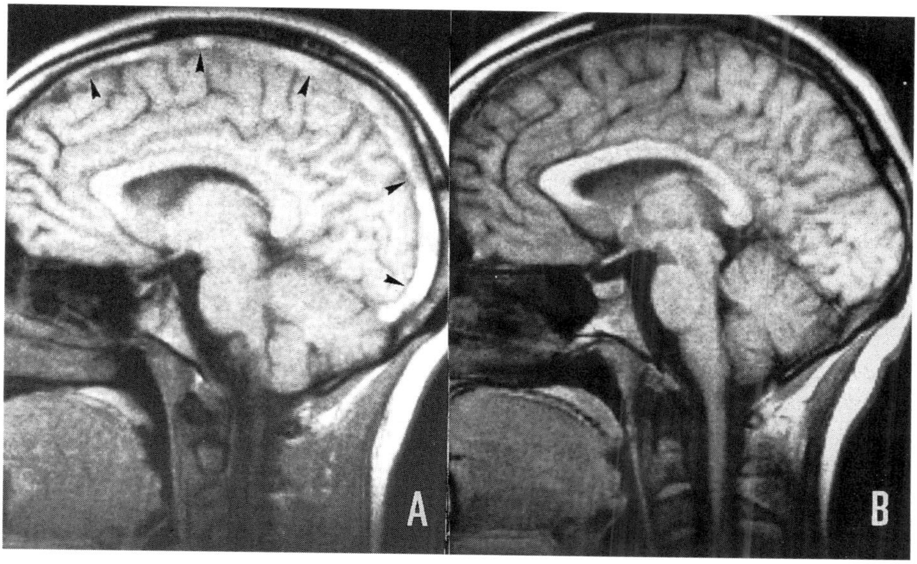

Figure 5.42 T1WI MRI showing SSS thrombosis at 3 weeks (A, arrows indicate increased signal) and at 3 months (B, normal).

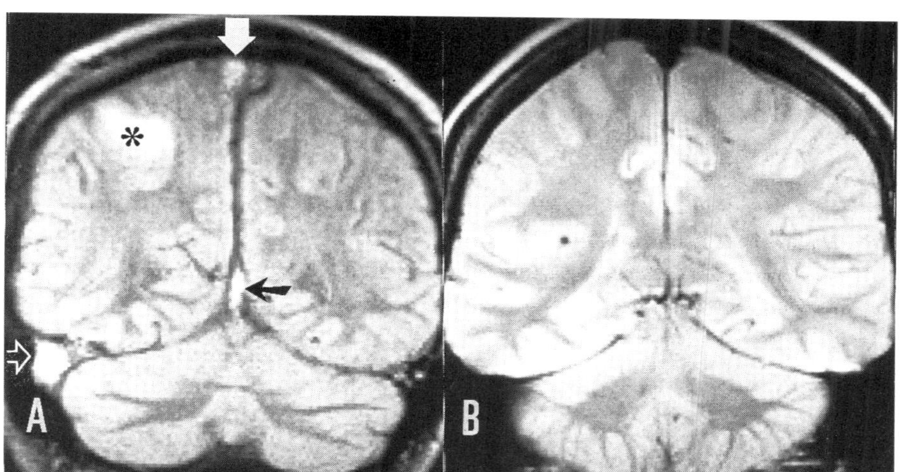

Figure 5.43 T2WI MRI showing extensive thrombosis of SSS (white arrow), straight sinus (black arrow) and left LS (open arrow) at 2 weeks (A, increased signal) and at 3½ months (B, normal). Parenchymal lesion with increased signal (asterisk) which is no longer seen 3½ months later (B).

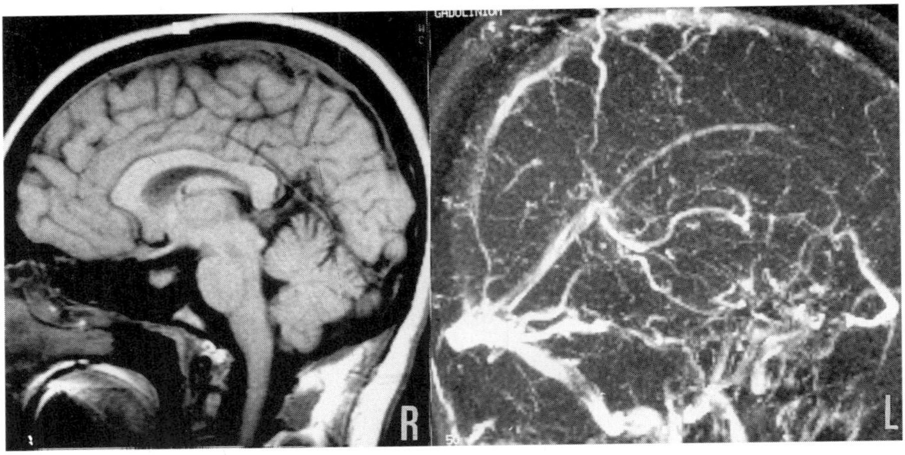

Figure 5.44 SSS thrombosis at 6 months with partial recanalization on T1WI MRI (R) and 2D TOF gadolinium-enhanced angiography (L).

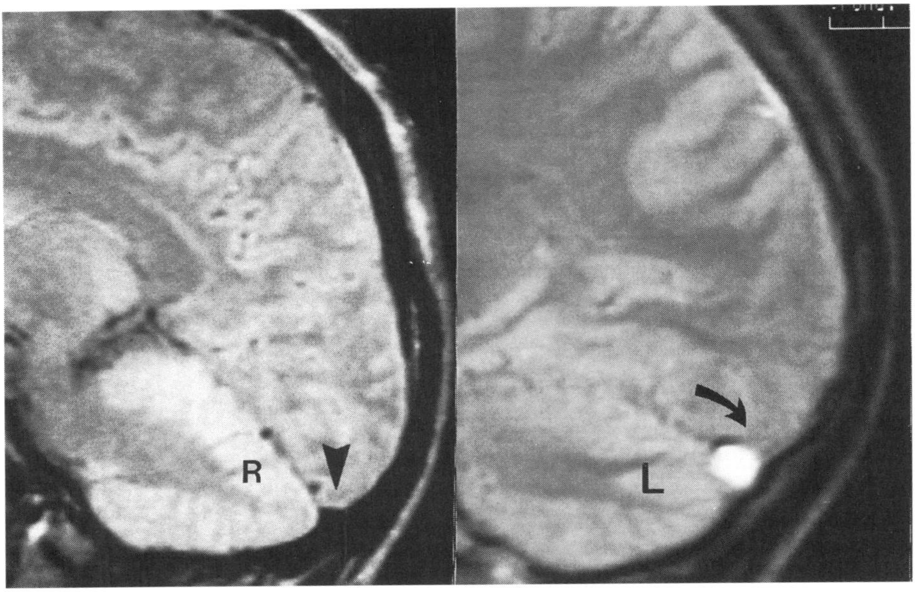

Figure 5.45 T1 parasagittal MR image of lateral sinus hypoplasia (R) and thrombosis (L) (indicated by arrows).

MRI is thus a remarkable tool in CVT in that it not only reveals the venous thrombosis but also illustrates the natural history of the thrombotic process. In a given patient, with occlusion of several sinuses, it indicates which sinus was affected first, sometimes giving a clue to the local cause. MRI is thus at present the method of choice for the diagnosis and follow up of CVT. MRI diagnosis is particularly easy in SSS thrombosis (Macchi *et al.*, 1986; Snyder and Sachdev, 1986; Thron *et al.*, 1986; Isensee *et al.*, 1994), but convincing images have also been obtained in cases of thrombosis involving LS (McMurdo *et al.*, 1986; Snyder and Sachdev, 1986; Mas *et al.*, 1990), straight sinus (Snyder and Sachdev, 1986), internal cerebral veins and the great vein of Galen (Hanigan *et al.*, 1986; Macchi *et al.*, 1986). MRI is particularly useful to differentiate thrombosis and hypoplasia of the LS. Mas *et al.* (1990) described six patients in whom angiography had shown non-visualization or poor visualization of one or both LSs. At MRI thrombosis appeared as an increased intraluminal signal on all planes and with all pulse sequences, whereas hypoplasia was characterized by a much smaller structure without any signal abnormality. This was best seen on parasagittal images, which allow the simultaneous identification of the triangular-shaped transverse portions of both lateral sinuses (Figure 5.45). Although MRI can also be useful for the diagnosis of cortical veins and cavernous sinus thrombosis (Savino *et al.*, 1986) (Figure 5.46), such cases remain notoriously difficult to diagnose, even with a combination of MRI and MRA.

Most MRI studies of CVT have been performed in adults, but similar changes have been reported in children and in newborn. Baram *et al.* (1988) described four cases of transverse sinus thrombosis in full-term infants who had an MRI 10–21 days after birth. All had an increased signal in the thrombosed sinus on both T1 and T2WI. Subdural and subarachnoid haemorrhages were associated, a frequent finding in the newborn but very rare in children and adults. MRI has recently been used successfully in larger series: that of Medlock *et al.* (1992), which included 11 neonates and two 5-year-old children; and that of Barron *et al.* (1992), which included 10 neonates and 15 children. MRI was considered 'superior to all other modalities for the diagnosis of CVT' in neonates and children. This is supported by Rivkin *et al.* (1992) who studied seven neonates with either lethargy or seizures caused by CVT, and found typical MRI appearances of increased sinus signal and absence of flow.

Gadolinium injection is generally of no use for the diagnosis of CVT. One should be aware that it induces signal changes opposite to those of the unenhanced thrombus. Circulating flow will appear as an increased signal and thrombosis as a decreased signal (Figure 5.47).

In some cases, interpretation of MRI in CVT is not easy because of false-negative and false-positive images (McMurdo *et al.*, 1986; Thron *et al.*, 1986; Sze *et al.*, 1988; Hulcelle *et al.*, 1989). False negatives are rare and mostly correspond to acute thrombosis studied in the first 2 or 3 days, to isolated cortical vein thrombosis or to cases studied too late, when sinuses have recanalized and are back to normal. In the series of 53 cases studies by Dormont *et al.* (1994), only

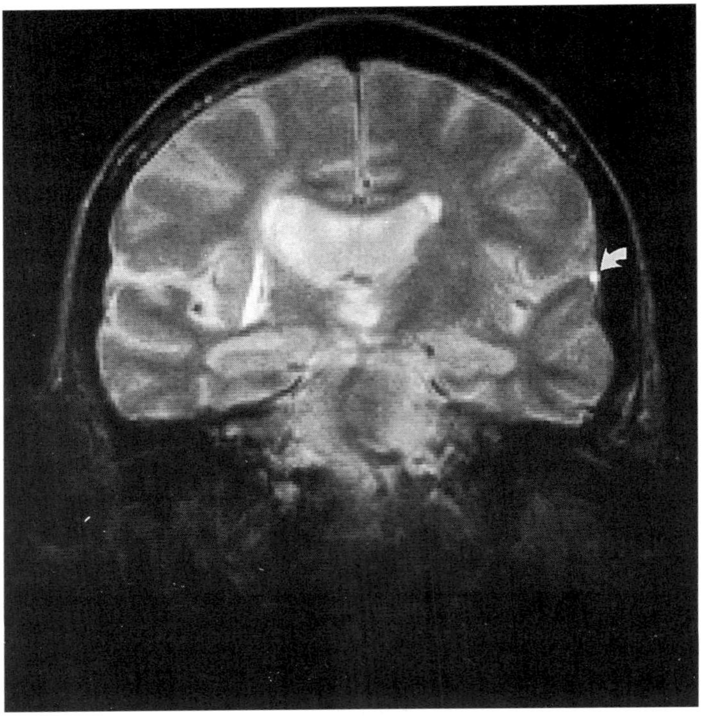

Figure 5.46 T2 MRI showing a hypersignal of an isolated cortical vein thrombosis (arrow) (the patient had a left deep middle central artery infarct some years before).

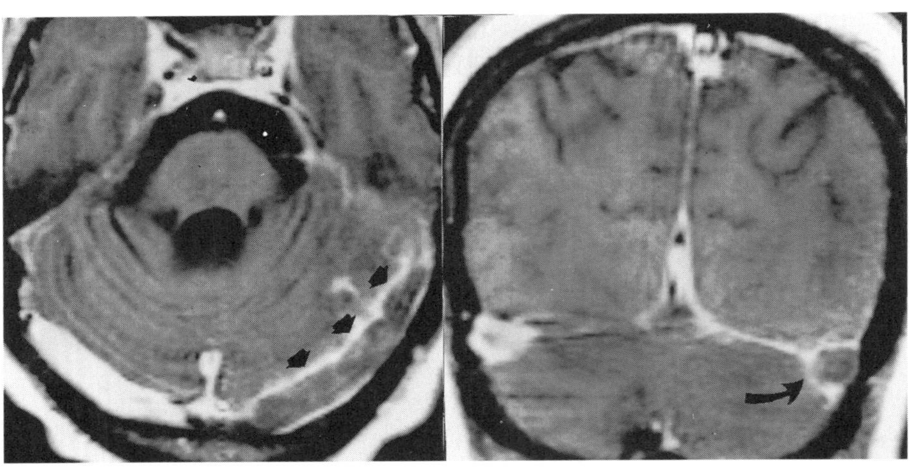

Figure 5.47 T1WI MRI with gadolinium, showing a decreased signal of the thrombosed right lateral sinus. Only the walls of the sinus are infected (arrows). The normal left LS shows a homogenous increase in signal.

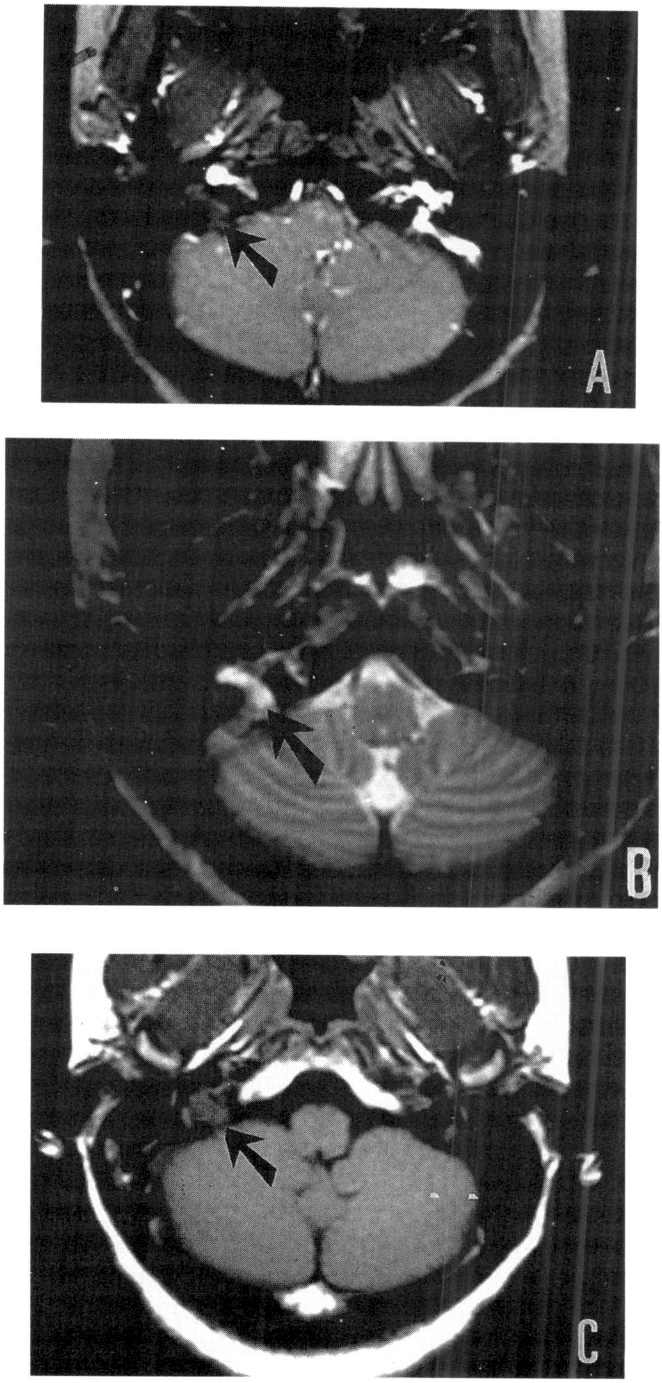
A
B
C

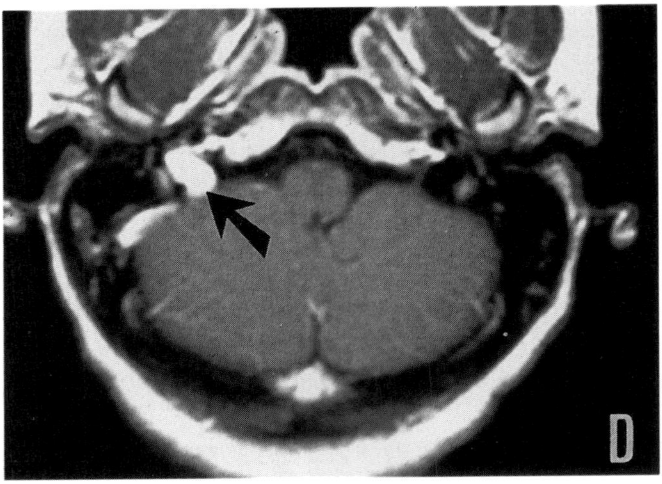

Figure 5.48 Axial MRI images of chronic (1 year) thrombosis of the left sigmoid sinus (indicated by arrows): (A) flow-sensitive frequency (GRASS) – no increased signal; (B) T2WI – increased signal; (C) T1WI – isosignal; (D) T1W1 with gadolinium – increased signal. (By courtesy of Dr D. Dormont, Neuroradiology Department, Pitié Hospital, Paris.)

three had normal MRI, two because of an isolated cortical vein thrombosis. In such cases, MRA is usually not sufficient and intra-arterial angiography is required in an attempt to detect the occluded artery or show the indirect signs of collateral circulation. False-negative images have also been reported with gadolinium-enhanced MR in chronic dural sinus thrombosis. Dormont *et al.* (1995) reported four patients with sinus thrombosis (SSS in three, LS in one) studied from 6 months to 2 years after the acute event. All had MRI signs of a chronic thrombus isointense on T1WI and hyperintense on T2WI. After injection of gadolinium, intense enhancement of the chronic thrombus was observed in all cases, undistinguishable from the adjacent normal sinuses (Figure 5.48).

False-positive images are infrequent, provided the appropriate sequences are used and the usual signal sinuses are known. The risk of false-positive images exists when the flow is severely slowed down, which happens, for instance, when there is a tumour invading a sinus. Three such cases have been reported by Daniels *et al.* (1989). The sinus patency was assessed by T1-weighted gradient echoimages and flow compensation, which confirmed the high signal intensity of patent sinuses. In certain cases, a false-positive increased signal can be observed in a small LS, probably owing to the existence of large temporal veins draining retrogradely. In such cases, slice orientations and sequences must be repeated to differentiate a true occlusion (constant signal abnormality in all projections) from a slow flow, which produces a signal varying with slice orientation.

PARENCHYMAL LESIONS

The patterns of parenchymal changes observed to date in CVT have been studied rarely on MRI, since the superiority of this technique over CT scan in that respect is less obvious than for the visualization of the thrombus itself. Brain swelling with mass effect and cortical sulcal effacement is the most frequent sign. It was found in 24 of the 256 cases reported by Yuh *et al.* (1994). Signal abnormalities are present in 60–70% of cases (Dormont *et al.*, 1994; Yu *et al.*, 1994). They most frequently consist of an increased signal in T2WI with a variable signal on T1WI (Figure 5.49): the increased T2 signal with an isosignal or hyposignal on T1 suggests interstitial oedema. In most cases there is no gadolinium enhancement, which suggests that this venous oedema is very different from the vasogenic oedema sometimes observed in arterial ischaemia (Yuh *et al.*, 1994). These lesions usually regress over a few weeks, which is another argument in favour of oedema rather than infarct (Figure 5.49).

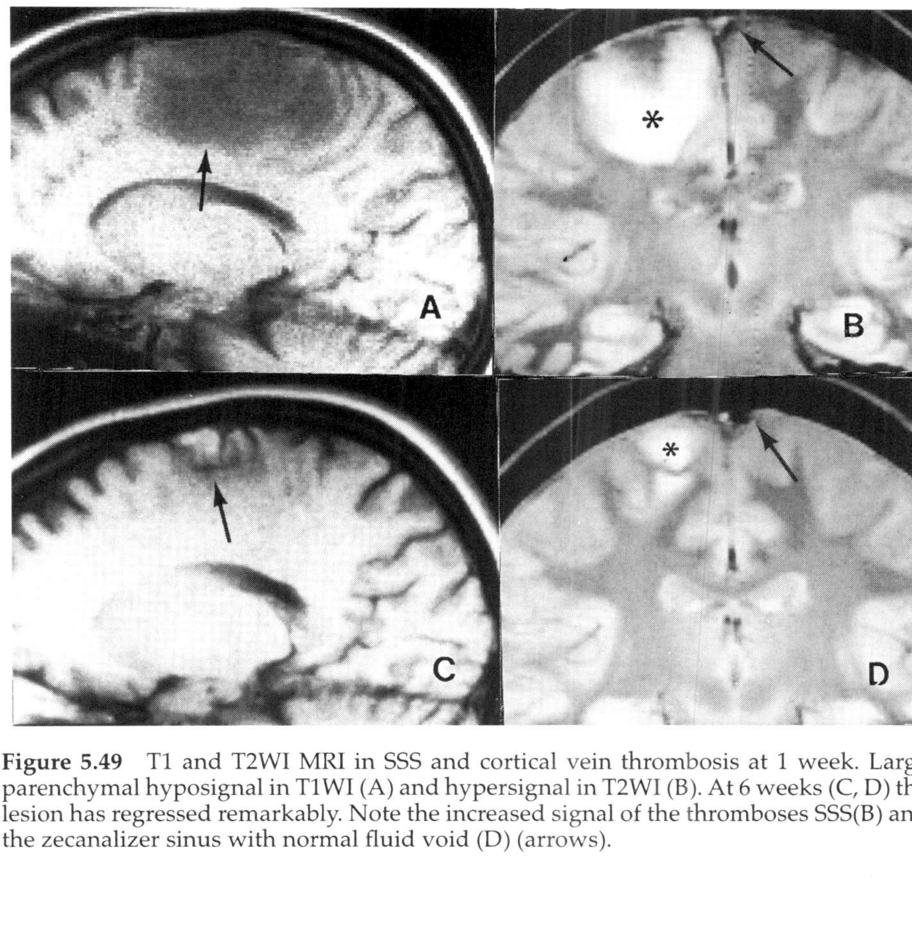

Figure 5.49 T1 and T2WI MRI in SSS and cortical vein thrombosis at 1 week. Large parenchymal hyposignal in T1WI (A) and hypersignal in T2WI (B). At 6 weeks (C, D) the lesion has regressed remarkably. Note the increased signal of the thromboses SSS(B) and the zecanalizer sinus with normal fluid void (D) (arrows).

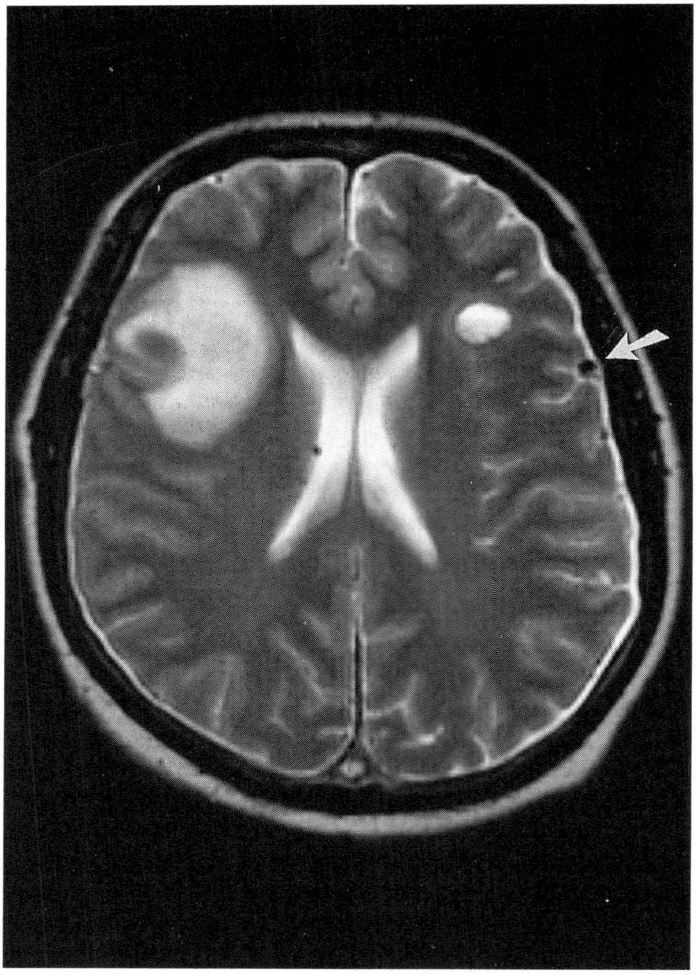

Figure 5.50 T2WI, MRI: SSS thrombosis with bilateral haemorrhages (a large one on the left, and two smaller ones on the right). Note the dilated cortical vein (arrow). (By courtesy of Dr B. Pertuiset, American Hospital, Paris.)

When there is a signal abnormality, in over half the cases [77% of Dormont's (1994) cases], there is a haemorrhagic component with an increased signal both on T1 and T2WI (Figure 5.50). This finding is slightly more frequent on MRI than on CT scan (Dormont *et al.*, 1994; Yuh *et al.*, 1994). Such a haemorrhagic component can be either petechial or a true haematoma with, on T2WI, a ring of decreased signal suggestive of haemosiderin. At a later stage, the whole lesion can appear as a hyposignal (Figure 5.51).

It has been suggested that these various MRI changes could be grouped in three distinctive patterns corresponding to different pathological changes (Yuh

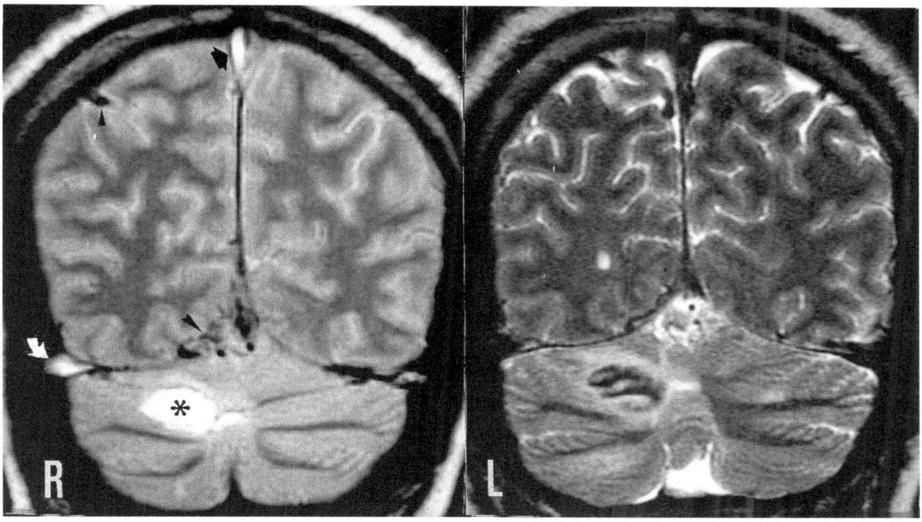

Figure 5.51 T2WI MRI showing thrombosis of the SSS (black arrows), left LS (white arrows) and cerebellar veins. Left cerebellar haemorrhage at 2 weeks (R) and at 4 weeks (L). (By courtesy of Dr B. Pertuiset, American Hospital, Paris.)

et al., 1994). The first pattern is brain swelling (sulcal effacement) without increased T2 signal. This corresponds to the distension of the venous bed without interstitial oedema. The second pattern is that of brain swelling with an increased signal on T2WI, which is likely to correspond to interstitial oedema. In the third pattern there is, in addition, the presence of blood. The location of parenchymal abnormalities depends on the site and extent of thrombosis. Bilateral parasagittal cortico-subcortical lesions are highly suggestive but usually appear late in the clinical course. Most often, there is a single lesion, which might be suggestive when it is a round or triangular cortex-based lesion in the frontal plane, and a round or oval lesion with an antero-posterior major axis in the axial or sagittal planes (Dormont *et al.*, 1994). These images are not specific but their diagnosis is easy because of the associated MRI signs of sinus thrombosis. The only difficulty is again with isolated cortical vein thrombosis. The parenchymal lesion can then be mistaken for a tumour unless there is a typical 'stop' sign with 'corkscrew' veins at angiography.

In conclusion, the combination of non-contrast MRI and MRA is nowadays the best method for the diagnosis and follow up of CVT. Its use is, however, limited in certain situations, such as a restless and confused patient or a deeply comatose subject requiring artificial ventilation in an intensive care unit. Unless there are contraindications, it should be performed as first-line investigation in case of high clinical suspicion. However, it requires: (1) a judicious use of all available spatial planes and of a variety of sequences; and (2) a perfect knowledge of the normal appearance of sinuses as well as of the various patterns of evolution of thrombosis. In the very rare normal or dubious cases, such as isolated cortical vein thrombosis, intra-arterial angiography may still be required.

OTHER INVESTIGATIONS

ELECTROENCEPHALOGRAM

Although it was extremely useful in the pre-CT scan era, the electroencephalogram (EEG) is nowadays of little interest in CVT because of the non-specificity of the changes observed, which mostly consist of a slow activity. Changes occur in roughly 75% of cases (Huhn, 1965; Burkhardt and Regli, 1974; Rao *et al.*, 1981; Bousser *et al.*, 1985; Rüttner, 1991). A generalized slow activity is described in up to 48% of all cases (Rao *et al.*, 1981; Bousser *et al.*, 1985; Rüttner, 1991). It is more frequent in patients with isolated intracranial hypertension than in those with focal signs, but it is then a useful sign, indicating a more diffuse impairment than clinically suspected (Bousser *et al.*, 1985). Focal slow activity may be seen in 15–24% of cases, almost exclusively in patients with focal clinical signs; signs of epileptic activity, e.g. sharp waves and spikes, are reported in 19% (Bousser *et al.*, 1985) to 33% (Burkhardt and Regli, 1964) of cases, mostly again in patients with focal clinical signs.

EEG is particularly useful in patients presenting with transient focal symptoms, to differentiate ischaemic and epileptic phenomena, and thus adapt the treatment accordingly. EEG can also be useful if it is abnormal in patients presenting with isolated headache. However, in 20–25% of cases, EEG is normal in CVT, particularly in patients presenting with isolated intracranial hypertension (Bousser *et al.*, 1985). In conclusion, there is no specific EEG pattern in CVT, but this investigation remains useful to point to an organic condition in patients presenting with isolated headache or to detect epileptic changes in patients with transient focal signs of undetermined nature.

ISOTOPE BRAIN SCANNING

Isotope brain scanning using technetium-99m- (Go *et al.*, 1973; Barnes and Winestock, 1977) or indium-111-labelled platelets (Bridgers *et al.*, 1986) has been shown to be helpful in identifying SSS and LS occlusion. However, some false negatives have been reported, probably owing to the visualization of an intense collateral circulation in the sinus walls. A case has been published of SSS thrombosis demonstrated by indium-111 platelet scintigraphy (Smith *et al.*, 1983). Early scintigraphy showed a focal increase in activity at each end of the thrombus, while later examination showed diffuse increase in activity in the sinus. Over the following 2 weeks platelet uptake declined markedly, thus giving information about the natural history of thrombosis. However, this technique is of no use in an emergency, since images are taken at 24 and 48 hours after injection, and it is no longer of practical importance since the development of MRI and MRA.

ULTRASOUND STUDIES

Very few studies have been devoted to ultrasound in CVT. Two cases of SSS thrombosis detected by sonography have been reported in the newborn (Edwards *et al.*, 1987), and some data have been published on the normal mean blood flow velocity in venous sinuses of newborns (Taylor, 1992) and adults (Aaslid *et al.*, 1982) using Doppler ultrasound. Recently transcranial Doppler has been used to detect SSS thrombosis in three patients. In the first case, Wardlaw *et al.* (1994) demonstrated a prominent venous signal adjacent to the middle cerebral artery away from the probe, which disappeared as the patient improved. There was, however, no control angiography. Valdueza *et al.* (1995) reported two angiographically confirmed examples of massive SSS thrombosis. Transcranial Doppler (TCD) detected a major increase in the mean blood flow velocity of basal veins probably corresponding to enlarged venous collateral pathways. If confirmed and extended, such results might have important practical applications, particularly because TCD is an inexpensive on-line method, which might allow day to day monitoring of those cases of SSS thrombosis that cannot be studied by MRI (Valdueza *et al.*, 1995).

CEREBROSPINAL FLUID EXAMINATION

Cerebrospinal fluid (CSF) examination is still a useful diagnostic tool in CVT because it is rarely entirely normal, in composition or in pressure: 10% in Ameri and Bousser's series (1992) and 26% in Barinagarrementeria *et al.*'s series (1992) (Garcin and Pestel, 1949; Kalbag and Woolf, 1967; Krayenbühl, 1967; Coquillat and Warter, 1976; Azzarelli *et al.*, 1980; Bousser *et al.*, 1985). In a majority of cases (40–60%), the pressure is increased and the composition is abnormal, but in a number of cases (up to 40%) (Barinagarrementeria *et al.*, 1992), there is an elevated pressure without alteration in the cytochemistry studies.

Abnormalities in composition include raised protein content in about half the cases, presence of red blood cells in two-thirds of cases and pleocytosis in one-third (Bousser *et al.*, 1985). The association of these three abnormalities is present in 30–50% of published cases and is thought to be highly suggestive. It is, however, in no way specific. The increase in protein is usually moderate (≤ 1 g l^{-1}) but occasionally the protein content can be as high as 3 or 4 g l^{-1}. Pleocytosis is also usually moderate (< 30 mm^3) with a preponderance of lymphocytes. However, a true meningitis is possible, either associated with the CVT or causal to it. The presence of a few red cells (< 20 mm^3) is frequent but sometimes difficult to differentiate from a traumatic lumbar puncture. On rare occasions, the amount of blood in CSF is sufficiently extensive to suggest subarachnoid haemorrhage from a ruptured aneurysm. Mainly found when focal signs are present, pleocytosis and the presence of red blood cells can also occur in patients presenting with 'benign intracranial hypertension' and the presence of these abnormalities should indicate sinus thrombosis as the possible cause of this syndrome (Bousser *et al.*, 1985). CSF examination is crucial in septic patients to rule out meningitis, which is extremely difficult to exclude on clinical grounds alone, in patients with symptoms of CVT.

Although in the era of CT and MRI, CSF study has become obsolete in the investigation of most non-septic CVT presenting with focal signs, it remains of the utmost importance in patients with isolated intracranial hypertension to rule out meningitis, to measure CSF pressure and to lower CSF pressure when vision is threatened. In such cases, it is therefore crucial to perform a lumbar puncture as early as possible, i.e. after the neuroimaging but before starting anticoagulation.

GENERAL INVESTIGATIONS

Having established the presence of CVT, investigations should be directed towards demonstrating the underlying aetiology. Because of the many causes, this is a long and difficult task. The presence of fever, of increased erythrocyte sedimentation rate or of raised polymorphonuclear cell count points to infective, inflammatory or malignant causes. However, even with such underlying diseases, these abnormalities are sometimes lacking and, conversely, they are occasionally found in idiopathic cases. Though rare, their presence is particularly useful to point to CVT in patients presenting with 'benign intracranial hypertension'. Investigations such as haematocrit, red blood cell count, platelet count, protid and lipid profile, and chest X-ray are systematically performed because they can lead to the detection of a variety of causes, such as polycythaemia vera, anaemia, thrombocythaemia, multiple myeloma, haemoconcentration, lung carcinoma or metastasis.

Detailed coagulation studies have only rarely been systematically performed in series of CVT and the results have been conflicting. Some have found a 'hypercoagulable state' (Poltera, 1972; Dindar and Platts, 1974) with an increase in platelet adhesiveness, aggregability and count (Bansal *et al.*, 1980), an increased fibrinogen (Srinivasan, 1983) and a decrease in fibrinolytic activity (Bansal *et al.*, 1980), but this was mainly during pregnancy and puerperium or in women taking oral contraceptives. Others did not confirm these results (Estanol *et al.*, 1979) or found as the only abnormality an increased platelet aggregation with the lowest dose of epinephrine (Bousser *et al.*, 1985). On the whole, there is no consistent abnormality that indicates the presence of a thrombotic process and the majority of CVT occur in the absence of these non-specific coagulation changes. The main interests of coagulation studies is thus not for the diagnosis of CVT but for the detection of possible causative conditions (Tarras *et al.*, 1988; Enevoldson and Ross Russell, 1990) such as protein C, protein S (Engesser *et al.*, 1987; Enevoldson and Ross Russell, 1990) or antithrombin deficiencies (Sauron *et al.*, 1982; Bousser *et al.*, 1985), antiphospholipid antibody syndrome (Levine *et al.*, 1987), essential thrombocythaemia

(Murphy *et al.*, 1983), or increased resistance to activated protein C (APC) (Svensson and Dahlbäck, 1994).

We have recently performed a systematic study of coagulation parameters (Deschiens *et al.*, 1996) in a series of 40 non-septic CVT patients, 29 with a known cause or predisposing factor other than a haematological disease, and 11 with an apparently idiopathic CVT. Coagulation abnormalities were found in six subjects: protein C deficiency in one, protein S deficiency in one and increased resistance to activated protein C with factor V Leiden mutation in four. Interestingly, there was only one case (protein S deficiency) without any other predisposing factor. The deficit in protein C was found in a patient with Behçet's disease, and the four cases of increased resistance to APC were, respectively, associated with nephrotic syndrome, systemic lupus erythematosus, antiphospholipid antibody syndrome and high doses of steroids in a patient with multiple sclerosis. Martinelli *et al.* (1996) found five cases of APC resistance with a point mutation (Arg 506) in the Factor V gene in a group of 25 patients with CVT who had no autoimmune, neoplastic or infectious disease. In four of these cases, there was another factor predisposing to CVT: oral contraceptives in two, puerperium in one and immobilization in one. Zuba *et al.* (1996) found the mutation in four of 19 patients with CVT (21%): in three of them, there was another prothrombotic factor: oral contraceptive use in two and puerperium in the third. Three other cases of CVT were reported in young women taking oral contraceptives and exhibiting APC resistence (Dulli *et al.*, 1996).

From these studies, it seems that APC resistance due to Factor V Leiden mutation may be the most frequent variety of thrombophilia underlying CVT. However, in most cases, CVT develops in the presence of a circumstantial acquired prothrombotic factor.

The inherited coagulation abnormalities are important to recognize because they often modify the long-term treatment and they imply a systematic family study. Thus, although they are infrequent causes, coagulation abnormalities should be looked for systematically in patients with CVT, whether or not there are other potentially causative factors, and particularly if there is a personal or family history of thrombotic venous disease. Coagulation tests should preferably be performed twice: the first one before the initiation of anticoagulant treatment and the second a few months after the acute episode. It is, however, possible to study proteins C and S while the patient is on heparin, and to study antithrombin and resistance to APC (Factor V Leiden) while on oral anticoagulants.

6

Outcome

SHORT-TERM OUTCOME

MORTALITY

Before the introduction of angiography, cerebral venous thrombosis (CVT) was mainly diagnosed at autopsy and, therefore, thought to carry a high mortality (Garcin and Pestel, 1949; Noetzel and Jerusalem, 1965; Kalbag and Woolf, 1967). In early angiographic series, this still ranged between 30% and 50% (Huhn, 1965; Krayenbühl, 1967). In a review of 203 cases reported between 1942 and 1990, Diaz *et al.* (1992) found an overall mortality of 49.3%. In more recent series, mortality rates have been highly variable, going from 6% (Ameri and Bousser, 1992) to 10–15% (Thron *et al.*, 1986; Virapongse *et al.*, 1987; Daif *et al.*, 1995), 23% (Barinagarrementeria *et al.*, 1992), and 38% (Rondepierre *et al.*, 1995). These discrepancies obviously reflect an important recruitment bias. It does remain true, however, that the outcome is far more favourable than originally thought, which explains the relatively low prevalence of CVT in autopsy studies.

There are three main causes of death in CVT. The first is the brain lesion itself, particularly when there is a massive haemorrhagic infarct, which can lead to herniation despite treatment for oedema. The second cause of death is intercurrent complications, such as sepsis, uncontrolled seizures and pulmonary embolism. In their review of 203 published cases, Diaz *et al.* (1992) found 23 cases with pulmonary embolism (11.3%) and, among these, the mortality rate was 95.6%. Such cases might indicate an underlying general hypercoagulable state but there are cases highly suggestive of direct propagation or embolization of the thrombus from the SSS to the pulmonary arteries via the jugular vein (Crimmins *et al.*, 1984; Diaz *et al.*, 1992). The third main cause of death is the underlying condition. Thus, in our series of 110 patients, there were six deaths, which all occurred in patients who had a severe underlying disease, such as subdural empyema, brain abscess, end-stage systemic lupus erythematosus and carcinomatous meningitis (Ameri and Bousser, 1992). In the recent series of Rondepierre *et al.* (1995) of 18 patients, two of the seven deaths were directly

Table 6.1 Outcome in recent series of patients with CVT

Outcome	Milandre *et al.* (1988)	Einhäupl *et al.* (1990)	Ameri and Bousser (1992)	Cantu and Barinagarrementeria (1993)		Tsai *et al.* (1995)	Daif *et al.* (1995)
				Puerperal	Non-puerperal		
	($n = 20$)	($n = 71$)	($n = 110$)	($n = 67$)	($n = 46$)	($n = 29$)	($n = 40$)
Total recovery	6 (30%)	42 (59%)	85 (77%)	36 (53.7%)	24 (52%)	22 (75.5%)	29 (72%)
Minor sequelae	8 (40%)	13 (18.5%)	11 (10%)	19 (28.3%)	3 (6%)	0	3 (8%)
Major sequelae	3 (15%)	6 (8.5%)	8 (7.5%)	6 (9%)	4 (9%)	1 (3.5%)	4 (10%)
Death	3 (15%)	10 (14%)	6 (5.5%)	6 (9%)	15 (33%)	6 (21%)	4 (10%)

related to the CVT (brain herniation), two were due to intercurrent complications and three were directly due to the underlying condition: lung carcinoma, septicaemia and paroxysmal nocturnal haemoglobinuria.

FUNCTIONAL RECOVERY

It has long been recognized that, if the patient survives the CVT, the prognosis for recovery of function is much better than in arterial thrombosis, with a minority (15–25%) of patients left with disabling sequelae (Coquillat and Warter, 1976; Bousser *et al.*, 1985; Thron *et al.*, 1986; Virapongse *et al.*, 1987; Milandre *et al.*, 1988; Barinagarrementeria *et al.*, 1992; Rondepierre *et al.*, 1995). Any combination of neurological signs can persist, according to the site, extent and severity of the parenchymal lesion, and to the degree of raised intracranial pressure. The most frequent sequels are blindness or lesser degrees of visual loss due to secondary optic atrophy, focal deficits (mainly motor or sensory), neuropsychological disturbances varying from mild memory disturbances or subtle behavioural changes to severe dementia usually of subcortical type, and seizures, which, as we will see later, are not frequent sequelae (Coquillat and Warter, 1976; Bousser *et al.*, 1985; Thron *et al.*, 1986; Virapongse *et al.*, 1987; Milandre *et al.*, 1988; Barinagarrementeria *et al.*, 1992; Rondepierre *et al.*, 1995). Some patients, particularly after deep cerebral venous system thrombosis or severe herniation, can remain severely disabled with quadriplegia, akinetic mutism or a persistent vegetative state. Some features are infrequent as sequelae of CVT, such as homonymous hemianopia, cerebellar incoordination and cranial nerve palsies (other than VIth). In neonates, the functional outcome mainly depends on associated illnesses. Thus in Shevell's (1989) series of 17 term neonates, neurologic development was normal in 11 of the 12 who had no asphyxia, whereas it was abnormal in 2 of the 4 who had CVT and asphyxia.

Such sequelae are now observed in a minority of cases and, in a number of recent series, there was a complete or near complete recovery in over 75% of cases: 77% in Ameri and Bousser's (1992) series, 78% in Einhäupl *et al.*'s (1990) series and 85% in a South African series (Hoffmann *et al.*, 1992). The pattern of recovery in CVT is remarkably different from that of arterial stroke. Even in patients with a severe and sometimes long-lasting deficit, improvement, when it occurs, can be very rapid. Some of our patients had a severe focal deficit for 1–3 weeks and suddenly regained normal function within 1 or 2 days.

PROGNOSTIC FACTORS

Numerous factors are thought to influence the prognosis of CVT.

Age

Age is one of the most important prognostic factors, with a high mortality rate in infancy and in the aged (Kalbag and Woolf, 1967; Towbin, 1973). As far as neonates are concerned, this was particularly true when severe dehydration, malnutrition, gastroenteritis and infection were frequent. A number of recent cases (Hanigan *et al.*, 1986; Baram *et al.*, 1988) and series (Shevell *et al.*, 1989; Barron *et al.*, 1992; Medlock *et al.*, 1992) suggest that the prognosis, though variable, is much better than previously thought. The prognosis seems to be good in term neonates presenting exclusively with seizures in the absence of systemic illness (Shevell *et al.*, 1989; Barron *et al.*, 1992; Medlock *et al.*, 1992). By contrast, outcome is still frequently unfavourable in premature neonates or when CVT is associated with other problems, such as asphyxia, shock or dehydration (Shevell *et al.*, 1989; Barron *et al.*, 1992). In older children, the most frequent mode of presentation is headache and the outcome is usually good (Barron *et al.*, 1992; Medlock *et al.*, 1992).

Clinical presentation

The clinical presentation is an extremely important prognostic factor: a rapid onset, the presence of coma and the presence of focal deficits (Garcin and Pestel, 1949; Krayenbühl, 1954; Kalbag and Woolf, 1967; Bousser *et al.*, 1985) are well-established factors for a bad prognosis. This issue has been specifically addressed in a recent series of 78 cases from Mexico (Barinagarrementeria *et al.*, 1992). Four clinical signs were statistically correlated with a poor prognosis: coma or stupor, bilateral pyramidal tract signs, generalized seizures, and meningeal signs. In another study of 77 patients, all those who were left with focal deficits or cognitive alterations as sequelae initially presented with focal signs (Preter *et al.*, 1996). By contrast, cases presenting with isolated signs of intracranial hypertension usually carry a good prognosis, provided the raised intracranial pressure is controlled. This should be done on an emergency basis to avoid herniation and visual loss owing to optic atrophy. The low death rate observed in our series is probably mainly explained by the high proportion (45%) of patients who presented with isolated intracranial hypertension.

Radiological signs

Radiological signs, such as the presence of a haemorrhagic infarct, an empty delta sign (Virapongse *et al.*, 1987) or bilateral lesions (Barinagarrementeria *et al.*, 1992) have been correlated with a poor prognosis.

Site of thrombosis

The site of thrombosis is a major prognostic factor, thrombosis of the deep venous system and of cerebellar veins carrying the worst prognosis and lateral sinus thrombosis the best. The classical picture of deep venous thrombosis was that of a rapidly lethal disease first presenting with headache, vomiting, impaired consciousness, hemiplegia or quadriplegia, and oculomotor disturbances (Ehlers and Courville, 1936; Bots, 1971; Averback, 1978; Eick *et al.*, 1981; Ur Rahman and Al-Tahan, 1993). The rare cases who survived were left with severe motor and neuropsychological disturbances (subcortical dementia). More recently, a number of cases have been reported with either minor sequelae

(Johnsen *et al.*, 1973; Nishimura *et al.*, 1982) or full recovery (Bousser *et al.*, 1985; Kim and Walczak, 1986; Haley *et al.*, 1989; Baumgartner and Landis, 1992). The same holds true for cerebellar vein thrombosis, which is exceedingly rare and has been mainly described at autopsy (Noetzel and Jerusalem, 1965). Some cases can, however, recover without sequelae (Bousser *et al.*, 1985; Rousseaux *et al.*, 1988).

Underlying condition

The underlying condition is a crucial prognostic factor. As already indicated, it is a major cause of death in CVT. Septic CVT remains a severe disease with a mortality rate of 30% in cavernous sinus thrombosis (DiNubile, 1988), 45% in cortical vein thrombosis (DiNubile *et al.*, 1990) and 78% in superior sagittal sinus (SSS) thrombosis (Editorial – *Lancet*, 1987). Other causes carrying a high risk of death are malignancies and blood disorders, particularly paroxysmal nocturnal haemoglobinuria (Van Vleymen *et al.*, 1987; Al Hakim *et al.*, 1993; Rondepierre *et al.*, 1995). By contrast, in old (Dubois, 1956; Stevens and Ammerman, 1965) as well as in recent series (Bansal *et al.*, 1980; Ameri and Bousser, 1992; Cantu and Barinagarrementeria, 1993), post-partum CVT seems to carry a relatively favourable prognosis, with complete recovery in 80 out of 129 cases in Srinivasan's (1983) series, in 100 out of 128 in Bansal *et al.'s* (1980) series and in 80% of the Mexican series. In these recent series, the death rate was about 10% (Bansal *et al.*, 1980; Cantu and Barinagarrementeria, 1993). Idiopathic cases have a variable outcome: in our series of 110 cases none died, whereas in the Mexican series 8 out of 20 patients died (Ameri and Bousser, 1992; Barinagarrementeria *et al.*, 1992).

VARIABILITY AND UNPREDICTABILITY OF PROGNOSIS

It is thus apparent that, although less severe than classically thought, the natural history and prognosis of CVT are highly variable. There are acute cases that can have a fulminating course leading to death in a few days, some who recover rapidly and completely, and others who are left with sequelae. There are chronic cases that worsen progressively leading to sequelae, whereas others recover spontaneously. There are extremely benign forms limited to transient ischaemic attack or headache, or epilepsy, which spontaneously recover and many are probably still unrecognized. On the whole, isolated sinus thrombosis carries a good prognosis, provided intracranial hypertension is controlled. However, sinus thrombosis can extend at any time to the cerebral veins and then possibly lead to death or sequelae, though only in a minority of cases.

A dramatic case has recently been reported, which illustrates this possibility of sudden worsening. A 30-year-old woman complained of sustained headaches and transient visual obscurations. Three months later, she suddenly became comatose, decerebrate and died within 48 hours of a massive deep venous system infarction (Ur Rahman and Al-Tahan, 1993). A prognostic scale has been proposed by Barinagarrementeria *et al.* (1992), based on clinical, computed tomography (CT) and cerebrospinal fluid (CSF) data. The presence of coma or of bilateral pyramidal signs rates as 3, that of generalized seizures rates as 2, and the presence of meningeal signs, bilateral lesions on CT scan and haemorrhagic CSF all rate at 2. These authors find a 100% good prognosis when the total score is ≤ 3 and a 100% bad prognosis when it is ≥ 9. The prognosis is usually good (85%) with a score of 4–5 and usually bad (90%) when the score is 6–8. However, applying this score to our series of 110 cases, we found two cases who had a score of 9 and yet made a complete recovery (Ameri and Bousser, 1992). Thus, although such a score is certainly an advance in the evaluation of prognosis, it should be validated in other series of CVT.

The prognosis is equally difficult to predict from the evolution of the thrombus. Although in lethal cases, extensive thrombosis of the involved vessels is the rule, there are a number of recent cases with persistent thrombosis or poor recanalization at magnetic resonance imaging who have made a complete recovery (Mas *et al.*, 1992). Thus, an early recanalization is an excellent prognostic sign but the absence of recanalization is not necessarily a poor prognostic sign.

In summary, although some clinical and radiological signs are correlated with a poor outcome, the prognosis for life as well as for disability remains extremely variable and largely unpredictable, which explains the difficulties and controversies about treatment.

LONG-TERM OUTCOME

DURAL ARTERIO-VENOUS FISTULA

Very little is known about the long-term outcome of patients with CVT. A few reports indicate that lateral sinus (LS) thrombosis can later induce the development of a dural arterio-venous fistula (Houser *et al.*, 1979; Bousser *et al.*, 1985; Graeb and Dolman, 1986; Mas *et al.*, 1992). Thus, in a series of 14 cases of arteriovenous malformations affecting the transverse sinus, 2 had angiographic evidence of sigmoid or transverse sinus occlusion, 1 and 4 years respectively, before the onset of symptoms related to the fistula (Houser *et al.*, 1979). The exact frequency of this late evolution of lateral sinus thrombosis is not known in the absence of prospective studies. It is, however, a rare complication: in our long-term study of 77 patients, there were 51 lateral sinus thrombosis and only one patient developed an arterio-venous fistula (Preter *et al.*, 1996). The relationship between these two conditions is a complex one because the spontaneous recanalization of a previous LS thrombosis can occur and in some cases coincide with the closure of the malformation, while in other cases the malformation persists (Kutluk *et al.*, 1991). In other cases, the arterio-venous fistula is pre-existent and can be the underlying cause of the LS thrombosis. This occurred in 3 out of our 51 cases of LS thrombosis (Preter *et al.*, 1996) and in 1 of the 10 cases reported by Enevoldson and Ross Russell (1990).

RISK OF RECURRENCE

The risk of recurrence of CVT is virtually unknown. In our series of 77 patients who were followed for a mean of 77.8 months, 9 (11.7%) suffered a recurrence, all but one in the first year (Preter *et al.*, 1996). Three of them had Behçet's disease, one had cancer and in the other five no aetiology could be found. Thrombotic events in other areas occurred in 11 subjects (14%), mainly in patients with a known cause, such as inflammatory diseases or thrombophilia. The risk of CVT recurrence during later pregnancies is an important practical issue on which there are only scanty published data. Srinivasan (1983) indicates that 5 out of 129 women became pregnant in the next 18 months and had a normal delivery without CVT recurrence. In our series, there were 16 pregnancies in 9 patients. Two of them had originally presented with pregnancy-related CVT. No uniform treatment was given (some had no treatment, some received heparin). No recurrence of CVT was observed during pregnancy or post-partum, regardless of the aetiology of the initial CVT, but one patient developed leg deep vein thrombosis during post-partum.

EPILEPSY

The incidence of epilepsy after CVT has been poorly evaluated. In one series of 19 patients (Nagpal, 1983), 6 later suffered from frequent epileptic seizures, whereas only 2 of the 20 patients reported by Milandre *et al.* (1988) had persisting seizures. In our series, seizures were rare: among the 28 patients who presented with seizures during the acute stage, only 4 had recurrent seizures during the follow-up period. They all had focal signs at the acute phase of the CVT, which again stresses the importance of focal signs as prognostic factors. Seizures occurred in the first year after the CVT (usually in the first few months) and were easily controlled with antiepileptic drugs (Preter *et al.*, 1996). No seizures occurred during the follow up in the 49 patients who did not have a seizure during the acute stage.

NEONATES

In neonates, very little is known about the long-term evolution of seizures, which are by far the most frequent mode of presentation of CVT. In their series of 17 neonates with CVT, Shevell *et al.* (1989) indicate that, among the 15 who presented with seizures, only 3 continued to have seizures beyond the neonatal period. It thus seems that the long-term prognosis of CVT-related epilepsy, in neonates as in adults, is relatively good, but precise data are very limited and further studies are needed to confirm these results.

LATE NEUROLOGICAL COMPLICATIONS

Late neurological complications (other than the sequelae of the initial event) virtually do not exist in CVT. One case has been reported of progressive dyskinesia developing in a 9-year-old boy 7 years after an internal cerebral vein thrombosis with bilateral thalamic lesions (Solomon *et al.,* 1982). One of our patients developed spasmodic torticolis 13 years after an extensive CVT, which involved cortical veins, cerebellar veins and the SSS.

In summary, although prospective data are lacking, it seems that the long-term prognosis of CVT is essentially good with a low rate of long-standing epilepsy, recurrent CVT and other thrombotic events.

7

Treatment

INTRODUCTION

As emphasized in the previous chapters, our knowledge of cerebral venous thrombosis (CVT) has changed completely in the last 20 years. Once thought to be invariably lethal, CVT now recovers without sequelae in the majority of cases. The classical clinical presentation was the association of a bilateral or alternating hemiparesis with seizures and disorders of consciousness, whereas we are now aware of the wide diversity of clinical presentations, from isolated headache, deficits or seizures to the most complex combinations of symptoms and signs. The presence of a haemorrhagic infarct was thought to be a constant feature, whereas it is now well established that this occurs in less than half the cases, the majority having either a normal brain on CT scan, or a hypodensity suggesting oedema or ischaemia. Most cases in the past were of infective origin, whereas nowadays, at least in developed countries, such an aetiology is rare.

We now know that this infrequent condition is extremely variable in its clinical presentation, mode of onset, imaging appearance and outcome, and that the prognosis remains largely unpredictable. It is thus not surprising that neurologists, the majority of whom have little experience of this condition, have not reached a consensus about treatment, particularly as far as the use of anticoagulant are concerned. Given the diversity of symptoms and causes, the three main arms of treatment, symptomatic, antithrombotic and aetiologic, should be decided on an individual basis.

SYMPTOMATIC TREATMENT

The two main features that treatment must address are seizures and raised intracranial pressure.

ANTICONVULSANTS

There is no disagreement concerning the use of anticonvulsants for CVT patients with seizures, whatever the type and number. Any of the major drugs can all be used and some recommend intravenous phenytoin to be started as rapidly as possible after the first seizure (Villringer *et al.*, 1994). The only point that is still debated is whether such treatment should be given to all patients or only to those who experience seizures. Kalbag and Woolf (1967) indicate that 'therapy should not await the onset of convulsions but should be used from the onset as prophylaxis . . . because of the importance of anoxic cerebral damage in major convulsions'. This opinion is shared by Einhäupl and Masuhr. (1994) who also think that, since seizures can induce necrosis, they should be systematically prevented. Chopra and Banerjee (1989) recommend prophylactic anticonvulsants when the EEG shows epileptic activity and also during the last trimester of pregnancy, and puerperium in patients with a previous history of CVT. Others, like us (Ameri and Bousser, 1992), prefer to restrict the use of anticonvulsants to patients who experience seizures.

The question of the duration of treatment remains open. As indicated above, long-term epilepsy is uncommon after CVT and there has been no study specifically devoted to this issue. In our series (Preter *et al.*, 1996), treatment was continued for 1 year in all patients who had seizures at the acute stage. It was later gradually discontinued in patients who had no recurrent seizures and a normal electroencephalogram (EEG). The late reappearance of seizures is extremely rare, and suggests either a recurrence of CVT or the presence of an underlying cause, which might have been overlooked.

METHODS TO REDUCE INTRACRANIAL PRESSURE

Raised intracranial pressure is a major adverse prognostic factor in CVT, both as regards the risk of death from brain herniation and the risk of blindness secondary to optic atrophy. Here again, treatment must be individualized. Like Einhäupl and Masuhr (1994) we do not treat the minor brain swelling that is observed in the majority of patients with CVT because it is well established that heparin treatment improves the venous outflow sufficiently to reduce intracranial pressure in most patients. When severe intracranial hypertension is present, other means should be used to reduce the pressure. A wide variety of methods have been used: corticosteroids, mannitol, fluid restriction, glycerol, dextran, acetazolamide or diuretics (Coquillat and Warter, 1976; Rousseaux *et al.*, 1978; Halpern *et al.*, 1984; Bousser *et al.*, 1985; Thron *et al.*, 1986; Feldenzer *et al.*, 1987; Einhäupl and Masuhr, 1994), lumbar punctures (Coquillat and Warter, 1976; Rousseaux *et al.*, 1978; Bousser *et al.*, 1985; Feldenzer *et al.*, 1987), ventricular cerebrospinal fluid (CSF) drainage (Feldenzer *et al.*, 1987; Hanley *et al.*, 1988), lumbo-peritoneal shunting (Bousser *et al.*, 1985; Ruel *et al.*, 1986; Engesser *et al.*, 1987), barbiturate-induced coma (Goldberg *et al.*, 1986; Feldenzer *et al.*, 1987; Hanley *et al.*, 1988), lateral sinus venous bypass (Sindou *et al.*, 1980), and even surgical decompression with or without removal of a haematoma (Ray and Dunbar, 1951; Krayenbühl, 1967; Buchanan and Brazinsky, 1970; Gettelfinger and Kokmen, 1977; Rousseaux *et al.*, 1978; Nagpal, 1983; Halpern *et al.*, 1984; Fevrier *et al.*, 1987).

The choice among all these methods depends on the individual clinical situation: steroids, such as dexamethasone, are often used and even sometimes considered as the drug of choice (Chopra and Banerjee, 1989). However, their efficacy is unproven and they should preferably be avoided (unless they are indicated to treat the underlying cause), because of their prothrombotic potential and the elevation of glucose and lactate concentration in the ischaemic brain (Einhäupl and Masuhr, 1994).

When patients present with isolated intracranial hypertension, and no brain lesion at CT scan or MRI we favour one lumbar puncture with sufficient fluid removal to obtain a normal closing pressure, before starting heparin. Such treatment (together with acetazolamide) is usually sufficient to improve headache and vision rapidly (assessed by the careful monitoring of visual fields, particularly the blind spot size, visual acuity and papilloedema). For the treatment of headache, paracetamol is the best choice; aspirin should be avoided owing to the increased haemorrhagic risk in conjunction with heparin. If vision continues to deteriorate (which in our experience is very rare), mannitol is added. Such a conservative approach is sufficient in the vast majority of cases. Some patients, particularly if treated late, may, however, require either further lumbar punctures or shunting procedures, or an optic nerve fenestration (Enevoldson and Ross Russell, 1990), but these treatments require a temporary interruption of heparin, which carries a risk of thrombosis progression. This was illustrated by one of our patients who presented with isolated intracranial hypertension. Owing to persistent transient visual obscurations, he had a few hours interruption of heparin for a repeat lumbar puncture, and just before lumbar puncture was performed, he experienced a massive left hemiplegia from extension of the superior sagittal sinus (SSS) thrombosis to a Rolandic vein, with a large non-haemorrhagic infarct on CT scan.

In patients with focal deficits and raised intracranial pressure, we and Einhäupl's group recommend the use of intravenous 20% mannitol (together with heparin) (Villringer *et al.*, 1994). This proves sufficient in the vast majority of cases. In resistant cases, intracranial pressure monitoring is necessary and other more drastic methods, such as lumbo-peritoneal shunting or barbiturate induced coma might be required (Feldenzer *et al.*, 1987; Hanley *et al.*, 1988).

Surgery has occasionally been performed to remove a localized intracerebral haematoma and to reduce intracranial pressure (Krayenbühl, 1967; Nagpal, 1983). In Nagpal's (1983) series of 80 patients, 34 underwent surgery when medical measures had failed and a large mass effect persisted as indicated by coma, unequal pupils and bradycardia. Of the 34 patients, 14 died following surgery, 18 were improved and 2 remained unchanged. Although it cannot be denied that surgery may have been life saving in some of these patients, the overall results do not seem to favour a surgical approach, which should generally be avoided because of its frequent harmful effect on a swollen and eventually haemorrhagic brain (Krayenbühl, 1967; Coquillat and Warter, 1976; Rousseaux *et al.*, 1978; Di Rocco *et al.*, 1981; Halpern *et al.*, 1984).

ANTITHROMBOTIC TREATMENT

ANTICOAGULANTS

Although the use of anticoagulants (heparin followed by warfarin) in CVT was first advocated more than 50 years ago (Martin and Sheehan, 1941; Stansfield, 1942), some authors are still sceptical about its value (Kaplan *et al.*, 1991; Stam *et al.*, 1991; Stam, 1993), for two main alleged reasons, the risk of intracerebral bleeding and the lack of evidence of efficacy.

Risk of intracerebral bleeding

The risk of intracerebral bleeding has been emphasized by a number of authors (Garcin and Pestel, 1949; Barnett and Hyland, 1953; Buchanan and Brazinsky, 1970; Gettelfinger and Kokmen, 1977; Rousseaux *et al.*, 1978), but rarely on the basis of undisputable evidence of a worsening directly related to the use of anticoagulants.

Barnett and Hyland (1953) were strongly against anticoagulants: 'we again want to emphasize the great danger in the use of anticoagulant therapy which has been advocated by most recent writers on this subject'. This was based on an autopsy series of 39 cases collected in 20 years, in which the authors were impressed by the haemorrhagic nature of the infarctions and the possible occurrence of massive subarachnoid haemorrhage.

Garcin and Pestel (1949) had previously made the same observations but they were not so negative. They said that anticoagulants should be used only with 'extreme caution' and 'might be deleterious in post-partum-related CVT because of the risk of uterine haemorrhage'.

Buchanan and Brazinsky (1970) likewise insisted that 'once focal neurologic signs have developed, the risk of haemorrhage militates against the use of anticoagulants' but this was not based on the two cases they reported, who were not anticoagulated.

Gettelfinger and Kokmen (1977) recommended that 'anti-coagulants should not be used in the therapy of SSS thrombosis'. This was based upon a series of seven cases, three of whom received anticoagulants and the other four did not. Two of the anticoagulated patients died while the other five made an uneventful recovery. The two fatal cases are worth reviewing briefly. The first one was a 27-year-old woman who had deep vein thrombosis 5 days before delivery. She was treated with heparin but developed thrombocytopenia, which led to the discontinuation of heparin. Two days post-partum, she had started to complain of severe headache, which persisted, associated with intermittent confusion after the discontinuation of heparin. Cerebral angiography performed a few days later disclosed SSS thrombosis and extensive thrombosis of deep and superficial veins bilaterally. Heparin was started again and, the next day, two infusions of urokinase were given. One hour after the second dose, she developed a right hemiplegia with incoherent speech due to a massive haemorrhage confirmed at autopsy. This is thus a very debatable case because, firstly, the patient had heparin-induced thrombocytopenia and, secondly, she was given urokinase, which seemed to be the immediate cause of the intracerebral bleeding.

The second case is equally difficult to interpret because it occurred in the setting of paroxysmal nocturnal haemoglobinuria, in a 33-year-old woman who was receiving subcutaneous heparin for pelvic vein thrombosis and antibiotics for endometritis. Two days later she experienced a sudden coma with right hemiparesis due to SSS thrombosis with a large intracerebral haematoma, which led to death. This case shows that heparin did not prevent CVT, a well-established fact in nocturnal paroxysmal haemoglobinuria (Johnson *et al.*, 1970; Ross, 1982; Van Vleymen *et al.*, 1987). Rousseaux *et al.* (1978) indicate without further details that they use heparin with extreme caution and only in cases devoid of venous infarcts because, in three of their cases, they observed 'a transformation of a venous infarct into a lethal intracerebral haemorrhage'.

Because of the paucity of undisputed cases of heparin-induced worsening in CVT, the case against its use for fear of intracerebral bleeding cannot therefore be regarded as proven and it seems that this potential risk has been overestimated. This is confirmed by the large number of cases and series in which anticoagulants have been given without deleterious effect. After the pioneer observations of Martin and Sheehan (1941) and Stansfield (1942), Krayenbühl (1954, 1967) was one of the strongest advocates of the use of heparin. In his series of 73 cases, 17 cases were treated with heparin and no intracerebral haemorrhage was observed. He noted that mortality was 7% in patients treated with anticoagulants and antibiotics, 37% in those treated with antibiotics only and 70% in those who received neither. He stated that he had never personally seen a patient with CVT who developed intracerebral haemorrhage during well-controlled anticoagulant treatment. Numerous other similar reports followed (Greitz and Link, 1966; Kalbag and Woolf, 1967; Fairburn, 1973; Castaigne *et al.*, 1977; Halpern *et al.*, 1984; Bousser *et al.*, 1985; Thron *et al.*, 1986; Einhäupl *et al.*, 1991; Ameri and Bousser, 1992; Einhäupl and Masuhr, 1994; Villringer *et al.*, 1994b). In our first series of 23 heparin-treated patients, there was no worsening and all suvived, 19 of them without sequelae (Bousser *et al.*, 1985). This series has been prospectively extended to 82 patients (Ameri and Bousser, 1992) all treated with heparin without any ill effect.

If most authors now agree that heparin is not dangerous in CVT patients with normal CT or with a hypodense lesion, many still believe that it is contraindicated in the presence of a haemorrhagic lesion on CT scan (Kalbag and Woolf, 1967; Rousseaux *et al.*, 1978; Gates, 1986). Yet there are now a number of cases of heparin treatment in CVT with haemorrhagic infarcts without any harmful effect (Halpern *et al.*, 1984; Bousser *et al.*, 1985; Goldberg *et al.*, 1986; Hosley *et al.*, 1991; Jackson *et al.*, 1993; El Koussa *et al.*, 1994). This has been confirmed on larger series of patients: 3 in Einhaupl *et al.*'s (1991) series, 4 in Milandre *et al.*'s (1988) series and 16 in our series (Ameri and Bousser, 1992). There are thus more than 30 reported cases of CVT with haemorrhagic infarcts, which have been treated with heparin without deleterious effect. It thus seems that in the evaluation of the risk–benefit ratio of heparin, the dangers of intracerebral bleeding have been greatly overestimated.

Efficacy of anticoagulants

Lack of evidence of efficacy is the second argument put forward by those who are sceptical about the use of anticoagulants in CVT. If only the results of large randomized trials are considered as evidence of efficacy, then it can be argued that evidence for heparin is slim because it is based on only one randomized study of 20 patients. However, many other observations militate in favour of anticoagulants, such as illustrative case reports and retrospective series.

A number of well-documented cases has been reported in which a dramatic improvement occurred after the initiation of heparin in patients who had previously been steadily deteriorating (Greitz and Link, 1966; Fairburn, 1973; Castaigne *et al.*, 1977; Halpern *et al.*, 1984; Bousser *et al.*, 1985; Thron *et al.*, 1986). There are four such cases in our series, two of them being particularly instructive.

The first was a 69-year-old woman who developed a right brachial monoplegia within a few hours (Castaigne *et al.*, 1977). She was apathetic, but not confused or dysphasic. She was given oral glycerin and dexamethasone but she deteriorated progressively. Her deficit extended to the leg, with a massive hemiplegia, she became dysphasic and then comatose. Nuclear brain scan (it was before the CT scan era) showed an increased uptake in the left fronto-Rolandic region and angiography showed a filling defect in the SSS with some cortical veins stopping abruptly before reaching the SSS. She was given high-dose heparin 20 days after the onset of symptoms when she was comatose with a dense right hemiplegia. Only 24 hours after starting heparin, she regained consciousness and within 10 days she could walk with support. She did not move her arm at all until the 20th day after the start of treatment but within the next 2 weeks she recovered completely.

Another dramatic improvement was observed in one of our patients who presented with left hemiplegia, headache, seizures and haemorrhagic infarct on CT scan. Because of this haemorrhage, heparin was considered to be contraindicated. The patient worsened and went into coma with bilateral extensor plantar response. CT scan revealed bilateral subcortical haemorrhages. It was then felt that the prognosis was so poor that there was nothing to lose. Heparin was started and within 48 hours the patient regained normal consciousness. Within 5 days she started to move her left hand and she made a full recovery within 2 weeks. Other cases are also very instructive in that patients improved with high-dose heparin, worsened when heparin was changed to oral anticoagulants or low-dose heparin, and rapidly improved again after full-dose heparin therapy was resumed (Fairburn, 1973; Thron *et al.*, 1986; Hosley *et al.*, 1991). The case reported by Hosley was that of a 26-year-old woman who had a SSS thrombosis post-partum with a slightly haemorragic infarct on CT scan. She improved on heparin but her headache relapsed when heparin was switched to oral anticoagulants with extension of thrombosis to the lateral sinus and jugular bulb. She improved again when heparin was resumed and made a complete recovery. Although the value of single case reports is limited, it is impressive to see that the number of well-documented cases of dramatic improvement shortly after initiation of heparin treatment exceeds by far the number of documented cases of haemorrhagic complications.

Heparin has been used since 1941 in many cases and series (Greitz and Link, 1966; Krayenbühl, 1967; Atkinson *et al.*, 1970; Fairburn, 1973; Coquillat and Warter, 1976; Rousseaux *et al.*, 1978; Halpern *et al.*, 1984; Bousser *et al.*, 1985; Thron *et al.*, 1986; Levine *et al.*, 1988; Einhäupl *et al.*, 1991; Ameri and Bousser, 1992; Einhäupl and Masuhr, 1994; Rondepierre *et al.*, 1995). Diaz *et al.* (1992) reviewed 203 CVT cases reported between 1942 and 1990, and compared the outcome of patients treated (54) and not treated (149) with heparin: 91% survived in the first group compared to 36% in the second. This would seem to be a strong argument in favour of anticoagulants, but it is of limited value because, in many of these cases, heparin was not given to patients who were comatose or had CT evidence of haemorrhagic infarcts. Such a bias has been emphasized recently by Stam *et al.* (1991) and Stam (1993) in a series of 62 cases in which the apparent benefit of heparin disappeared when comatose patients (who had been denied heparin) were excluded from the analysis. This, however, is not the case in Einhäupl *et al.*'s (1991, 1994) and in our series (Ameri and Bousser, 1992), where heparin has been used during the last 10 years whatever the clinical presentation and the CT image, with favourable results. Thus, in Einhäupl *et al.*'s (1991) series, among the 27 patients with intracranial haemorrhage who received heparin, 4 died (15%) compared with 9 out of 13 who did not receive heparin (69%). A complete recovery was observed in 14 heparin-treated patients (51%) and in 3 (23%) of the untreated group. In the German and French series combined (Villringer *et al.*, 1994), 143 patients received heparin. Only four of them died; they had in common an extremely rapid progression of the disease and were comatose when heparin treatment was started.

Such good results are, however, still difficult to interpret because it is highly probable that neuroimaging facilities now allow earlier diagnosis and that we are treating more benign cases, which previously might have recovered spontaneously. It has long been known and it is widely documented that CVT can recover spontaneously even when haemorrhagic infarcts are present (Garcin and Pestel, 1949; Kalbag and Woolf, 1967; Krayenbühl, 1967; Coquillat and Warter, 1976; Estanol *et al.*, 1979; Bansal *et al.*, 1980; Bousser *et al.*, 1985; Milandre *et al.*, 1988; Cantu and Barinagarrementaria, 1993). This seems to be particularly so in neonates who are rarely treated with anticoagulants (Shevell *et al.*, 1989; Barron *et al.*, 1992; Medlock *et al.*, 1992). The exact frequency of such spontaneous recovery is not known but it has certainly been underestimated in the past. Such a good outcome is more frequent in patients who present with isolated intracranial hypertension than in those who have focal signs and parenchymal lesions on CT scan, but there are cases of patients with coma or with bilateral haemorrhagic infarcts who recover with only symptomatic treatment. Such cases are, however, totally unpredictable and, as strongly emphasized by Kalbag and Woolf (1967): 'in sinus thrombosis, the patient is in danger of cerebral infarction at any moment from spread of thrombosis to the cerebral veins', as illustrated by a number of cases (Bousser *et al.*, 1985; Feldenzer *et al.*, 1987; Ur Rahman and Al-Tahan, 1993).

Only one randomized study of heparin treatment in CVT has so far been reported (Einhäupl *et al.*, 1991). The investigators had planned to include 60 patients and performed an interim analysis after the first 20 patients. The interim analysis was considered so positive in favour of anticoagulants that the study was discontinued early. Twenty patients with angiographically proven sinus venous thrombosis were randomly allocated either to dose-adjusted intravenous heparin or to placebo. The dose of heparin was an initial bolus of 3000 IU and then 25 000–65 000 IU each day, adjusted to double the initial activated partial thromboplastin time (PTT), but not to exceed 120 seconds (target 80–100 seconds). At the start of treatment three patients in the heparin group and two in the placebo group had haemorrhage on CT scan. The outcome measures were the results of a specially designed severity scale and the development of intracerebral haemorrhage at CT scan, which was performed at least twice. The clinical course of the two groups started to diverge in favour of the heparin group after 3 days of treatment ($p < 0.05$) and the difference remained significant ($p < 0.01$) after 8 days of treatment. After 3 months, eight of the heparin-treated patients had a complete clinical recovery and two had only slight residual neurologic deficits. This contrasts with the placebo group in which only one patient had a complete recovery, six had neurologic deficits and three died ($p < 0.01$). In the group treated with heparin, complications included haematuria, a groin haematoma, and a stillbirth but no new brain haemorrhage. Among the three patients who had intracerebral haemorrhage before treatment, two made a complete recovery. In the placebo group, one patient died of pulmonary infarction, three had new brain haemorrhages, two of whom did not have haemorrhage at onset. Although the methodology of this trial has been criticized, particularly as regards the use of a non-validated severity scale, the results are impressively in favour of heparin. Some authors consider them as only 'encouraging' and have started a double-blind multicentre trial comparing low-molecular-weight heparin and placebo, and aiming at recruiting 30 patients in each group (Stam, 1993).

Another argument in favour of heparin treatment is the risk of pulmonary embolism, during the acute phase of CVT, which was well recognized in the past but widely overlooked until the work of Diaz *et al.* (1992), who found 23 cases (11.3%) in their literature review of 203 cases and reported a case of their own. Of these 23 cases, 22 died and the only survivor had been on anticoagulation therapy. Pulmonary embolism is thus a dramatic complication of CVT, which might be prevented by the use of heparin.

Indication for anticoagulants

From the above review of literature, there is good evidence that the risk–benefit ratio of heparin in CVT is favourable, but there is also good evidence that a number of patients with CVT can recover without the use of heparin. This explains the divergent opinions about the best indications of heparin. All agree that heparin is indicated in patients with coexistent pelvic or deep leg vein thrombosis and pulmonary embolism, but such cases are a minority. Others advocate the use of anticoagulants when there is evidence of 'extension of the cerebral lesion at CT monitoring' (Chopra and Banerjee, 1989). However, this position seems difficult to hold since, as we have seen, CT is not a sensitive investigation to assess the extension and propagation of the thrombotic process. A still widely held view is that anticoagulants are indicated provided there is no haemorrhage on CT scan (Kalbag and Woolf, 1967; Gettelfinger and Kokmen, 1977; Estanol *et al.*, 1979; Sigsbee *et al.*, 1979; Gates, 1986; Feldenzer *et al.*, 1987; DiNubile, 1988; Kaplan *et al.*, 1991). However, an increasing number of authors are in favour of anticoagulants, even in patients with a haemorrhagic infarct (Halpern *et al.*, 1984; Bousser *et al.*, 1985; Milandre *et al.*, 1988; Einhäupl *et al.*, 1991; Ameri and Bousser, 1992; Jackson *et al.*, 1993; Einhäupl and Masuhr, 1994; Koussa *et al.*, 1994; Rondepierre *et al.*, 1995).

At one stage, when the risk of intracerebral bleeding was still overestimated, we recommended the use of heparin only when patients deteriorated despite symptomatic treatment (Castaigne *et al.*, 1977; Bousser *et al.*, 1985), and this is still the policy of some authors (Barinagarrementeria *et al.*, 1992; Cantu and Barinagarrementaria, 1993). Such an attitude certainly allows a number of cases to recover spontaneously but it does not face the problem of sudden extension of thrombosis, and it delays the use of heparin until there is a major brain lesion, a situation in which heparin might be more deleterious. We are thus faced with a dilemma: either treat all patients knowing that this treatment is probably unnecessary in a number who would have spontaneously recovered, or restrict treatment to those who worsen despite symptomatic treatment, knowing that it will be too late for some patients and that it will carry a higher risk of intracerebral bleeding. Since, firstly, it is impossible to predict which patients are going to recover spontaneously and which will suddenly worsen, and, secondly, the risk of anticoagulants is low and even more so when there is no or minimal brain lesion, we have adopted the following policy [which is also that of the German group (Einhäupl *et al.*, 1991; Einhäupl and Masuhr, 1994; Villringer *et al.*, 1994)] in the last 10 years. Our policy is to anticoagulate with heparin all patients with demonstrated CVT, irrespective of the clinical presentation and of the CT findings, provided there is no general contraindication to the use of heparin (Ameri and Bousser, 1992; Bousser and Barnett, 1992). This applies to adults and children, but not to neonates where most authors agree that anticoagulation appears unnecessary (Barron *et al.*, 1992; Rivkin *et al.*, 1992).

The value of heparin has also been discussed in relation to the aetiology of CVT. Some authors have suggested that heparin is contraindicated in septic CVT because the risk of intracranial bleeding is increased and because the thrombus might help confine the infection, thus preventing dissemination of septic emboli with subsequent miliary abcesses (Karlin and Robinson, 1984; Shaw, 1952; Smith, 1984; Southwick *et al.*, 1986). However, these risks are very poorly documented and should be weighed against the benefit of treatment. There is no randomized study specifically devoted to septic CVT, but Levine *et al.* (1988) reviewed 134 cases of cavernous sinus thrombosis from 1910 to 1985 and compared those treated with antibiotics alone (82) with those treated with a combination of antibiotics and anticoagulants (52), dividing this last group into those with early (16) and late (36) anticoagulation. They found no conclusive evidence for reduction of mortality with the combination but they showed that early anticoagulation reduced morbidity (blindness, stroke, ophthalmoplegia, hypopituitarism and focal seizures). Complications of anticoagulant therapy were rare and the authors concluded that anticoagulants were indicated early in the treatment of cavernous sinus thrombosis. Although it is clear that the first treatment of septic CVT is antibiotics, the available evidence is again in favour of adding heparin to antibiotics.

There is not much debate about the indication for heparin when there is an underlying general disease with an increased thrombotic tendency, such as Behçet's disease (Wechsler *et al.*, 1992), systemic lupus erythematosus (Vidailhet *et al.*, 1990), or a congenital thrombophilia, such as protein C, protein S or antithrombin III deficiencies (Enevoldson and Ross Russell, 1990; Confavreux *et al.*, 1994). By contrast, the use of heparin is controversial in paroxysmal nocturnal haemoglobinuria. Some consider it as a contraindication because of the frequent presence of thrombocytopenia, the increased risk of haemorrhage, the inability to prevent thrombosis in other areas (Gettelfinger and Kokmen, 1977; Van Vleymen *et al.*, 1987) and the possibility of spontaneous recovery (Benoit *et al.*, 1986). Others indicate that 'if the patient develops CVT, the only available treatment is anticoagulation' (Al Hakim *et al.*, 1993), particularly since some patients have improved with heparin (Rondepierre *et al.*, 1995). There is no specific treatment for this severe condition. Some have indicated the use of androgen but such treatment might also induce thrombosis (Shiozawa *et al.*, 1982). It is, therefore, impossible to give firm recommendations about the use of heparin in this disease. In our series, there was only one patient affected. She developed isolated intracranial hypertension with massive papilloedema and multiple transient visual obscurations. A lumbar puncture was performed to remove some CSF and heparin treatment was immediately started, with an uneventful recovery.

Anticoagulation modalities

The initial anticoagulant treatment of CVT is essentially similar to that of deep vein thrombosis in the legs (Weinmann and Salzman, 1994). Heparin is the drug of choice, given with either a continuous intravenous infusion or with subcutaneous injections. These modalities are preferable to intermittent intravenous injections, which increase the risk of bleeding. Most authors favour the infusion route (Einhäupl *et al.*, 1991; Villringer *et al.*, 1994) but its superiority to the subcutaneous administration has not been established. For deep vein thrombosis of the legs, the two routes are equally effective provided the activated partial thromboplastin time is maintained in the prescribed therapeutic range (2–2.5 times the control value) (Einhäupl *et al.*, 1991; Villringer *et al.*, 1994).

The optimal duration of heparin is not established. For deep vein thrombosis, a regimen of 5 days of heparin followed by oral anticoagulants is regarded as conventional therapy but, in CVT, a more prolonged treatment is advocated because of the occasional reports of worsening when heparin was switched to oral anticoagulants (Fairburn, 1973; Thron *et al.*, 1986; Hosley *et al.*, 1991). There is no fixed duration of treatment but, empirically, heparin is usually prolonged until the patient improves or at least stabilizes (Villringer *et al.*, 1994). If the patient improves rapidly, oral anticoagulants should be started early since the shorter the heparin treatment, the less often it is followed by heparin-induced thrombocytopenia. By contrast, heparin should be maintained in pregnancy-related CVT because of the risk of oral anticoagulants during pregnancy. Caution is also required in patients with homozygous protein C and S deficiencies because of the risk of haemorrhagic skin necrosis induced by oral anticoagulants if the patient is not fully anticoagulated with heparin prior to starting warfarin (Samama *et al.*, 1984).

Low-molecular-weight heparin might prove as effective as conventional heparin but there is so little experience in CVT (Fevrier *et al.*, 1987) that heparin should at present be preferred.

In most cases, after a few days, heparin is switched to warfarin adjusted to obtain an international normalized ratio (INR) between 2 and 3. There are no controlled data on the required duration of oral anticoagulation but in Einhäupl *et al.*'s (1991) prospective study there was no recurrence of CVT after 3 months. This is the usually recommended duration of treatment (Ameri and Bousser, 1992; Villringer *et al.*, 1994), particularly when there is a known acute cause without risk of prolonged thrombotic tendency, such as minor head trauma, post-partum or local infection. By contrast, prolonged treatment is warranted whenever there is a continuing risk of thrombosis, such as lengthy immobilization, malignant disease, inflammatory disease (Behçet's disease, systemic lupus, etc.), inherited thrombophilia or recurrent venous thrombosis.

The following case illustrates the risk of recurrent venous thrombosis after stopping anticoagulant treatment in a patient with inherited thrombophilia. A 32-year-old man experienced grand-mal seizures followed by a left hemiplegia. Brain CT scan showed a right Rolandic haemorrhagic infarct, and magnetic resonance imaging (MRI) disclosed SSS thrombosis. The patient was treated with antiepileptic drugs and heparin, and rapidly switched to oral anticoagulants. He recovered rapidly and, since no cause was found, oral anticoagulants were stopped 4 months later. Within a few days, he developed deep vein thrombosis of the legs and pulmonary embolism from which he recovered. Factor V Leiden was then detected, which later proved to be familial.

The attitude towards anticoagulant treatment during later pregnancies in women who had previous CVT is not clear because very few data have been reported. If there is a known underlying prothrombotic tendency, preventive heparin should be used. In other cases, there are two approaches: either systematic heparin treatment, or no treatment, but an extremely close follow up with appropriate investigations and treatment at the earliest suspicion of CVT. Some of our patients had uneventful pregnancies either with or without treatment. Our attitude is now to use preventative heparin treatment when the initial CVT occurred during pregnancy and in patients who have a history of recurrent venous thrombosis. In other cases we recommend close follow up. For women who had post-partum CVT, we favour the immediate use after delivery of low-dose prophylactic heparin for one month (Bousser, 1996).

OTHER ANTITHROMBOTIC TREATMENTS

Antiplatelet drugs

The risk of promoting intracranial bleeding with heparin has led some authors to suggest the alternative use of aspirin or dipyridamole in CVT (Gettelfinger and Kokmen, 1977; Estanol *et al.*, 1979; Chopra and Banerjee, 1989; Yerby and Bailey, 1980). This attitude has never been properly evaluated and seems illogical, since antiplatelet drugs are of no proven value in the acute treatment of venous thrombosis or pulmonary embolism, although they may have some prophylactic efficacy (Antiplatelet Trialists' collaboration, 1994). Furthermore, they also carry an increased risk of haemorrhage.

Thrombolytic treatment

Vines and Davis (1971) were the first to report on the use of thrombolytic treatment in CVT. They studied 10 patients with sinus thrombosis and relied on retrograde jugular venography as a diagnostic tool. Five patients were treated with intravenous urokinase but details of treatment are not given. One patient worsened, three gradually improved and one made a dramatic recovery. Angiography did not show major changes after treatment. After two rather negative reports (each based on a single case) (Gettelfinger and Kokmen, 1977; Rousseaux *et al.*, 1978), Di Rocco *et al.* (1981) recommended the combination of intravenous urokinase infusion with heparin for 2–6 days. This regimen was applied to five patients (four with SSS thrombosis, one with lateral sinus thrombosis), who all recovered uneventfully and showed sinus patency at angiography. Since these pioneer reports, thrombolytic treatment has been used in some 50 cases, either locally or intravenously (Scott *et al.*, 1988; Higashida *et al.*, 1989; Persson and Lilja, 1990; Barnwell *et al.*, 1991; Eskridge and Wessbecher, 1991; Medlock *et al.*, 1992; Tsai *et al.*, 1992; van Dyke *et al.*, 1992; Griesemer *et al.*, 1994; Smith *et al.*, 1994; Horowitz *et al.*, 1995).

In 1988, Scott *et al.* reported a single case of extensive SSS thrombosis treated with a local urokinase infusion via a frontal burr hole. The patient, who was initially decerebrate, made a good recovery despite the occurrence of a haemorrhagic infarct a few hours after the beginning of the infusion.

In 1989, Higashida *et al.* treated a transverse sinus thrombosis in a newborn child by direct sagittal sinus puncture and instillations of 12 000 units of urokinase over a 12-hour period. The thrombus cleared and the child remained neurologically normal 3 years later. In 1990, Persson and Lilja performed an open thrombectomy and instilled urokinase into the SSS. Despite formation of a cerebellar haematoma, the patient gradually improved but did not completely recover. In 1991 and 1992, Barnwell *et al.* and Tsai *et al.* reported three and five patients, respectively, from the same institution, all treated with transvenous catheterization and urokinase instillation. Seven of the eight patients had a good recovery and none had complications related to therapy. Smith *et al.*, in 1994, reported a series of seven patients who failed a trial of medical therapy and were also treated with direct infusion of urokinase, via the femoral route in one patient and the internal jugular route in six. Patency of the occluded sinus (SSS in two, lateral sinus in five) was achieved in all cases and the patients improved. A series of 13 patients has recently been reported by Horowitz *et al.* (1995). They all had extensive sinus thrombosis involving SSS in 12, lateral sinus in 12 and straight sinus in 4. They were all treated with local urokinase infusion via the transfemoral route. Sinus patency was obtained in 12 out of 13 patients and good to excellent clinical outcome was also achieved in 12 patients. The authors conclude that the effectiveness of fibrinolytic therapy in sinus thrombosis is demonstrated. It should, however, be remembered that all these reports on thrombolytics in CVT were uncontrolled, that heparin was usually given with and after thrombolytic treatment, that in the majority of cases (Horowitz *et al.*, 1995) no other treatment had been adequately tried before thrombolysis, and that a number of CVTs can recover spontaneously. It is thus extremely difficult to evaluate properly the effectiveness of this therapeutic approach.

The risk of thrombolytic treatment in CVT is equally unknown. The above-mentioned authors all conclude that it is a safe method, but only a few patients with haemorrhagic infarcts have been treated so far. These were excluded in Smith *et al.*'s (1994) series of 7 patients, and only 4 of the 13 patients studied by Horowitz *et al.* (1995) had a haemorrhagic infarct.

These preliminary studies are thus insufficient to assess the risk–benefit ratio of thrombolytic treatment in CVT properly. They have confirmed that dural sinus venography is feasible, and they have shown that local urokinase infusion is possible and is effective in recanalizing the thrombosed sinus. This is in keeping with what is known in other areas, where thrombolytic treatment with streptokinase or recombinant tissue plasminogen activator, followed by anticoagulation is more effective than anticoagulation alone for the restoration of patency of a thrombosed vein (Weinmann and Salzman, 1994). However, the clinical effectiveness of thrombolytics in CVT needs to be confirmed on larger series. As far as the risks are concerned, there is no doubt that thrombolytics induce a two-fold to four-fold increase in the risk of intracranial bleeding when given for deep venous thrombosis of the leg or for myocardial infarction. They are thus likely also to carry an increased risk of intracerebral bleeding in patients with CVT.

From these preliminary data, it is difficult to come to any conclusions on thrombolytic therapy in CVT. Although results are promising, we still favour the use of heparin because of its good results established on a much wider experience and because of its lower risk of intracerebral bleeding. There is, however, a case for trying local thrombolysis in patients worsening despite symptomatic treatment and adequate heparin anticoagulation, and there might also be a case for a randomized trial to compare these two treatment regimens. However, such a trial would have to be a very large multicentre study given the low frequency of this condition and the variability of its prognosis.

Surgical ligation and thrombectomy

Tying of the jugular vein was once used in septic lateral sinus thrombosis. It was thought to be effective in isolating the septic source in the lateral sinus from the general circulation and in preventing thromboembolism (Cody, 1939). Others disagreed and emphasized that this procedure was often followed by septic complications, and could promote retrograde thrombosis and increase intracranial hypertension by interrupting the venous drainage (Lyman, 1935; O'Connell, 1990). Internal jugular vein ligation is no longer performed in the treatment of CVT. The surgical removal of thrombi in SSS was performed by Ray and Dunbar in 1951. Interestingly the patient did well, although the venogram 6 weeks later showed that the sinus was blocked as before but that an anastomotic circulation had developed. Estanol *et al.* (1979) recommended thrombectomy in patients with rapid visual loss or dangerous intracranial pressure despite symptomatic treatment. They recognized that surgery should not be done for cortical vein thrombosis or when there was a haemorrhagic infarction. The risk of surgery on a swollen and sometimes haemorrhagic brain has been emphasized by many authors (Krayenbühl, 1967; Coquillat and Warter, 1976; Rousseaux *et al.*, 1978; Di Rocco *et al.*, 1981) and there is now little support for this method of antithrombotic treatment.

AETIOLOGICAL TREATMENT

Whenever possible, the cause of the CVT should be treated on its own merits, in association with symptomatic treatment and anticoagulation. This applies particularly to septic thrombosis, which still carries a high mortality and should be treated with a wide-spectrum combination of antibiotics, associated in some cases with the surgical treatment of the primary site of infection, such as surgical drainage of paranasal, middle ear or mastoid infections (DiNubile,

1988). The choice of the antimicrobial drug will obviously depend on the causative agent, the results of culture, the primary site of infection, and the presence or absence of other infectious complications, such as meningitis or septicaemia. A combination of a penicillinase-resistant penicillin with a third-generation cephalosporine and metronidazole has been advocated as appropriate empirical therapy in septic cavernous sinus thrombosis (DiNubile, 1988). The exact duration of antibiotics will depend on the clinical response, the primary site of infection and the presence of associated complications, but often exceeds 2 weeks. Surgery is sometimes necessary to treat the primary site of infection, such as middle ear, sinusitis, dental abscess or brain abscess. The optimal timing of surgery is not clear but it is probably better to operate on any primary focus of infection as early as possible (Editorial – *Lancet*, 1987; DiNubile, 1988).

As indicated in previous chapters, sepsis is no longer the first cause of CVT and the catalogue of causes is ever increasing. It is important to treat the underlying cause whenever possible because it influences both the immediate outcome (a number of deaths is at present directly related to the aetiology) and the long-term prognosis. Failure to recognize the cause might lead to CVT recurrence. This was the case in one of our patients who was first seen for internal cerebral vein thrombosis interpreted as idiopathic. She recovered spontaneously, but a year later she presented with SSS thrombosis and general signs of Behçet's disease (Bousser *et al.*, 1985).

SUMMARY

Treatment of CVT is based primarily on heparin, followed by warfarin, associated when necessary with symptomatic treatment (anticonvulsants and reduction of raised intracranial pressure) and, whenever possible, with an aetiological treatment, such as antibiotics in septic cases. Other modalities of antithrombotic treatment are at present anectodal.

References and further reading

Aaslid R, Markwalder TM, Normes H (1982) Non invasive transcranial Döppler ultrasound recording of flow velocity in basal cerebral arteries. *Journal of Neurosurgery* **57**: 769–774.

Abercrombie J (1828) *Pathological and Practical Researches on Diseases of the Brain and Spinal Cord*. Edinburgh: Carfrae & Son. pp. 83–85.

Abumiya T, Echizenya K, Ihara T, Murai H, Satou M (1992) A case of venous thrombosis associated with medullary venous malformation. *Neurological Surgery* **20**: 451–455.

Achiron A, Gornish M, Melamed E (1990) Cerebral sinus thrombosis as a potential hazard of antifibrinolytic treatment in menorrhagia. *Stroke* **21**: 817–819.

Agah R, Rice L, Winikates J (1996) Fatal cerebral venous thrombosis as the initial manifestation of the antiphospholipid syndrome. *Clinical Neurology and Neurosurgery* **98**: 189–191.

Akova YA, Kansu T, Dumas S (1993) Pseudotumour cerebri secondary to dural sinus thrombosis in neurosarcoidosis. *Journal of Clinical Neuro-ophthalmology* **13**: 188–189.

Al Hakim M, Katirji MB, Osorio I, Weisman R (1993) Cerebral venous thrombosis in paroxysmal nocturnal hemoglobinuria: report of two cases. *Neurology* **43**: 742–746.

Ambruso DR, Jacobson CJ, Hathaway WE (1980) Inherited antithrombin III deficiency in a child. *Pediatrics* **65**: 125–131.

Ameri A, Bousser MG (1992) Cerebral venous thrombosis. *Neurologic Clinics* **10**: 87–111.

Ameri A, Bousser MG (1993) Headache in cerebral venous thrombosis: a study of 110 cases. *Cephalalgia* **13** (Suppl 13): 110.

Aminoff MJ (1973) Vascular anomalies in the intracranial dura mater. *Brain* **96**: 601–612.

Anderson CM, Edelman RR, Turski PA (1993) Magnetic resonance venography and cerebral venous thrombosis. In: *Clinical Magnetic Resonance Angiography*, Vol. 1 (eds CM Anderson, RR Edelman and PA Turski), pp. 289–308. New York: Raven Press.

Anderson SC, Shah CP, Murtagh FR (1987) Congested deep subcortical veins as a sign of dural venous thrombosis: MR and CT correlations. *Journal of Computer Assisted Tomography* **11**: 1059–1061.

Andrew D (1865) Thrombosis of cerebral sinuses, with apoplexy of optic thalami, consequent on anaemia. *Transactions of the Pathology Society of London* **16**: 27–28.

Angelov A (1989) Intracranial venous thrombosis in relation to pregnancy and delivery. *Pathology Research and Practice* **185**: 843–847.

Antiplatelet Trialists' Collaboration (1994) Collaborative overview of randomised trials of antiplatelet therapy. III. Reduction in venous thrombosis and pulmonary embolism by antiplatelet prophylaxis among surgical and medical patients. *British Medical Journal* **308**: 235–246.

Anxionnat R, Blanchet B, Dormont D *et al.* (1994) Present status of computerized tomography and angiography in the diagnosis of cerebral thrombophlebitis cavernous sinus thrombosis excluded. *Journal of Neuroradiology* **21**: 59–71.

Askenasy HM, Kosary IZ, Braham J (1962) Thrombosis of the longitudinal sinus: diagnosis by carotid angiography. *Neurology (New York)* **12**: 288–292.

Ata M (1965) Cerebral infarction due to intracranial sinus thrombosis. *Journal of Clinical Pathology* **18**: 636–640.

Atkinson EA, Fairburn B, Heathfield KWG (1970) Intracranial venous thrombosis as a complication of oral contraception. *Lancet* **1**: 914–918.

Auer LM, Pucher R, Leber K, Ishiyama N (1987) Autoregulatory response of pial vessels in the cat. *Neurological Research* **9**: 245–248.

Averback P (1978) Primary cerebral venous thrombosis in young adults: the diverse manifestations of an underrecognized disease. *Annals of Neurology* **3**: 81–86.

Azzarelli B, Itani AL, Catanzaro PT (1980) Cerebral phlebothrombosis: a complication of lymphoma. *Archives of Neurology* **37**: 126–127.

Bailey OT, Hass GM (1937) Dural sinus thrombosis in early life, clinical manifestations and extent of brain injury in acute sinus thrombosis. *Journal of Pediatrics* **11**: 755–771.
Bank I, Weart C (1984) Dural sinus thrombosis in Behçet's syndrome. *Arthritis and Rheumatism* **27**: 816–818.
Banker BQ (1961) Cerebral vascular disease in infancy and childhood. 1. Occlusive vascular disease. *Journal of Neuropathology and Experimental Neurology* **20**: 127–139.
Bansal BVC, Gupta RR, Prakash C (1980) Stroke during pregnancy and puerperium in young females below the age of 40 years as a result of cerebral venous / sinus thrombosis. *Japanese Heart Journal* **21**: 171–183.
Baram TZ, Butler IJ, Nelson MD, McArdle CB (1988) Transverse sinus thrombosis in newborns: clinical and magnetic resonance findings. *Annals of Neurology* **24**: 792–794.
Barinagarrementeria F, Cantu C, Arredondo H (1992) Aseptic cerebral venous thrombosis: proposed prognostic scale. *Journal of Stroke and Cerebrovascular Disease* **2**: 34–39.
Barker GB (1949) Injuries to the superior longitudinal sinus. *British Medical Journal* **1**: 1113–1116.
Barnes BD, Winestock DP (1977) Dynamic radionuclide scanning in the diagnosis of thrombosis of the superior sagittal sinus thrombosis. *Neurology (New York)* **27**: 656–661.
Barnett HJM, Hyland HH (1953) Noninfective intracranial venous thrombosis. *Brain* **76**: 36–49.
Barnwell SL, Higashida RT, Halbach VV *et al.* (1991) Direct endovascular thrombolytic therapy for dural sinus thrombosis. *Neurosurgery* 1991, **28**: 135–142.
Barraquer-Bordas L, Bachs A, Barraquer-Moner J (1955) La forme subaigue de la thrombophlébite du sinus caverneux. *La Presse Médicale* **63**: 376–378.
Barré JA, Grenier C (1932) Etude clinique et anatomique d'un cas de thrombophlebite cérebrale-partielle puerpérale. *Revue Neurologique* **58**: 361–379.
Barron TF, Gusnard DA, Zimmerman RA *et al.* (1992) Cerebral venous thrombosis in neonates and children. *Pediatric Neurology* **8**: 112–116.
Batson OV (1940) Function of the cerebral veins and their role in the spread of metastases. *Annals of Surgery* **112**: 138–147.
Baumgartner RW, Landis T (1992) Venous thalamic infarction. *Cerebrovascular Disease* **2**: 353–358.
Bedford THB (1935) Effect of increased intracranial venous presure on pressure of CSF. *Brain* **58**: 427–447.
Belman AL, Roque CT, Ancona R *et al.* (1990) Cerebral venous thrombosis in a child with iron deficiency anaemia and thrombocytosis. *Stroke* **21**: 488–493.
Benoit P, Lozes G, Destée A, Jouet JP, Jomin M, Warot P (1986) Hypertension intracranienne bénigne et maladie de Marchiafava Micheli. *Revue Neurologique* **142**: 782–785.
Bloemenkamp KWM, Rosendaal FR, Helmerhorst FM *et al.* (1995) Enhancement by factor V Leiden mutation of risk of deep-vein thrombosis associated with oral contraceptives containing a third generation progestagen. *Lancet* **346**: 1593–1596.
Borda IT, Southern RF, Brown WF (1973) Cerebral venous thrombosis in ulcerative colitis. *Gastroenterology* **64**: 116–119.
Bots GAM (1971) Thrombosis of the galenic system veins in the adult. *Acta Neuropathologica* **17**: 227–233.
Bouchut JE (1879) Thrombose cachectique des sinus de la dure-mére et convulsions finales des maladies de l'enfance. *Gazette des Hopitaux Civils et Militaires* 52: 225–226, 258–259, 306–308, 395–396, 441–442, 603–605, 690–692, 764–766, 787–789.
Bousser MG (1993) Treatment of cerebral venous thrombosis. *Cerebrovascular Disease* **3**: 329–330.
Bousser MG (1996) Thromboses veineuses cérébrales. In: *Pathologies maternelles et grossesse*. Vol. 1, 2nd ed. (eds B Wechsler, J Janse-Marec, JC Pechere). Paris: McGraw Hill. (in press).
Bousser MG, Blétry O, Launay M *et al.* (1980) Thromboses veineuses cérébrales au cours de la maladie de Behçet. *Revue Neurologique* **136**: 753–762.
Bousser MG, Chiras J, Sauron B *et al.* (1985) Cerebral venous thrombosis. A review of 38 cases. *Stroke* **16**: 199–213.
Bradshaw P (1956) Benign intracranial hypertension. *Journal of Neurology, Neurosurgery and Psychiatry* **19**: 28–41.
Brant-Zawadzki M, Chang GY, McCarty GE (1982) Computed tomography in dural sinus thrombosis. *Archives of Neurology* **39**: 446–447.
Bresnan MJ, Strand R, Rosenbaum A (1973) Jugular venous thrombosis associated with benign intracranial hypertension. *Neurology* **23**: 390.
Bridgers SL, Strauss E, Smith EO *et al.* (1986) Demonstration of superior sagittal sinus thrombosis by indium-111 platelet scintigraphy. *Archives of Neurology* **43**: 1079–1081.

Brismar J (1980) Computed tomography in superior sagittal sinus thrombosis. *Acta Radiologica (Stockh)* **21**: 321–326.
Brookfield DSK (1974) A case of primary cerebral thrombosis. *Postgraduate Medical Journal* **50**: 767–768.
Brown MT, Friedman HS, Oakes WJ *et al.* (1991) Sagittal sinus thrombosis and leptomeningeal medulloblastoma. *Neurology* **41**: 455–456.
Brown P (1961) Septic cavernous sinus thrombosis. *Bulletin of the John Hopkins Hospital* **109**: 68–75.
Brunquell PJ, Rosenberger PB (1982) Recurrent cavernous sinus syndrome complicating supratentorial arteriovenous malformations. *Stroke* **13**: 865.
Buchanan DS, Brazinsky JH (1970) Dural sinus and cerebral venous thrombosis. Incidence in young women receiving oral contraceptives. *Archives of Neurology* **22**: 440–444.
Bucy PC, Lesemann FJ (1942) Idiopathic recurrent thrombophlebitis with cerebral venous thrombosis and acute subdural haematoma. *Journal of the American Medical Association* **119**: 402–405.
Buonanno F, Moody DM, Ball MR, Laster DW (1978) Computed cranial tomographic findings in cerebral sino-venous occlusion. *Journal of Computer Assisted Tomography* **2**: 281–290.
Buonanno F, Moody DM, Ball MR (1979) Radionuclide sinography diagnosis of lateral sinus thrombosis by dynamic and static brain imaging. *Radiology* **130**: 207–213.
Buonanno FS, Moody DM, Ball RM (1982) CT scan findings in cerebral sinovenous occlusion. *Neurology* **12**: 288–292.
Burkhardt S, Regli F (1964) EEG veranderungen bei 27 Fällen von zerebraler Thrombophlebitis. *Schweizer Archives Neurologie Neurochirurgie und Psychiatrie* **94**: 1–14.
Byers RK, Hass GM (1933) Thrombosis of dural venous sinuses in infancy and childhood. *American Journal of the Diseases of Childhood* **45**: 1161–1183.
Byrne JV, Lawton CA (1983) Meningeal sarcoidosis causing intracranial hypertension secondary to dural sinus thrombosis. *British Journal of Radiology* **56**: 755–757.
Cambria S (1980) Infarctus cérébral hémorragique par thrombose de la veine de Labbé. *Revue de Neurologie* **136**: 321–326.
Cantu C, Barinagarrementeria F (1993) Cerebral venous thrombosis associated with pregnancy and puerperium; review of 67 cases. *Stroke* **24**: 1880–1884.
Carroll JD, Leak D, Lee HA (1966) Cerebral thrombophlebitis in pregnancy. *Quarterly Journal of Medicine* **35**: 347–368.
Case Reports of the Massachussetts General Hospital (1960) *New England Journal of Medicine* **263**: 1080–1084.
Castaigne P, Laplane D, Bousser MG (1977) Superior sagittal sinus thrombosis. *Archives of Neurology* **34**: 788–789.
Caudill CM, French LA, Haines GL (1953) Increased intracranial pressure following compression of the superior sagittal sinus. *Neurology* **3**: 231.
Cavazos JE, Caress JB, Chilukin VR *et al.* (1994) Sumatriptan-induced stroke in sagittal sinus thrombosis. *Lancet* **343**: 1105–1106.
Cervos-Navarro J, Kannuki S (1990) Neuropathological findings in the thromboses of cerebral veins and sinuses: vascular aspects. In *Cerebral Sinus Thrombosis, Experimental and Clinical Aspects*, Vol. 1 (eds K. Einhaüpl, O. Kempski and A. Baethman), pp. 15–25. New York: Plenum Press.
Chakeres DW, Schmalbrock P, Brogan M *et al.* (1991) Normal venous anatomy of the brain: demonstration with gadopentetate dimeglumine in enhanced 3D MR angiography. *American Journal of Neuroradiology* **156**: 161–172.
Chelly D, Levy C, Ameri A, Brunereau L (1994) Imagerie des thrombophlébites cérébrales. *Annales de Radiologie* **37**: 108–117.
Chilvers E, Rudge P (1986) Cerebral venous thrombosis and subarachnoid haemorrhage in users of oral contraceptives. *British Medical Journal* **I**: 292–524.
Chiras J, Bousser MG, Meder JF *et al.* (1985) CT in cerebral thrombophlebitis. *Neuroradiology* **27**: 145–154.
Chiras J, Bousser MG, Dormont D *et al.* (1991) Thrombophlébites cérébrales. In *Imagerie du Système Nerveux*, Vol. 1 (eds F. Le Bras, A. Gaston, C. Marsault), pp. 388–397. Paris: Flammarion.
Chopra JS, Banerjee AK (1989) Primary intracranial sinovenous occlusions in youth and pregnancy. In: *Handbook of Clinical Neurology* (ed. JF Toole), Part II, pp. 425–452, Vascular Diseases, Vol. 10 (54). Amsterdam: Elsevier.
Chung JW, Chang KH, Han MH *et al.* (1988) Computed tomography of cavernous sinus diseases. *Neuroradiology* **30**: 319–328.
Clifford-Jones RE, Ellis CJK, Stevens JM, Turner A (1982) Cavernous sinus thrombosis. *Journal of Neurology, Neurosurgery and Psychiatry* **45**: 1092–1097.

Cobb S, Hubbard JP (1929) Cerebral haemorrhage from venous or capillary stasis. *American Journal of Medical Science* **178**: 693–709.
Cochran FB, Packman S (1992) Homocystinuria presenting as sagittal sinus thrombosis. *European Neurology* **32**: 1–3.
Cockerell OC, Lai HM, Ross Russell, RW (1993) *Pseudotumour cerebri* associated with arterio-venous malformations. *Postgraduate Medical Journal* **69**: 637–640.
Cody CC Jr (1939) Thrombosis of the lateral sinus. *Archives of Otolaryngology* **29**: 674–680.
Collier W (1891) Thrombosis of cerebral veins. *Lancet* **1**: 544.
Conard J, Horellou MH, Van Dreden P, Samama M (1987) Pregnancy and congenital deficiency of antithrombin III or Protein C. *Thrombosis and Haemostasis* **58**: 39 (abstract).
Confavreux C, Brunet P, Petiot P *et al.* (1994) Congenital Protein C deficiency and superior sagittal sinus thrombosis causing isolated intracranial hypertension. *Journal of Neurology, Neurosurgery and Psychiatry* **57**: 655–657.
Coquillat G, Warter JM (1976) Thromboses veineuses cérébrales. Rapport de neurologie présenté au *Congrès de Psychiatrie et de Neurologie de Langue Française*, Vol. 1, Paris: Masson Ed.
Corbett JJ, Mehta MP (1983) Cerebrospinal fluid pressure in normal obese subjects and patients with pseudotumor cerebri. *Neurology* **33**: 1386–1388.
Crawford SC, Digre KB, Palmer CA *et al.* (1995) Thrombosis of the deep venous drainage of the brain in adults. Analysis of seven cases with review of literature. *Archives of Neurology* **52**: 1101–1108.
Crimmins TJ, Rockswold GL, Yock DH Jr (1984) Progressive posttraumatic superior sagittal sinus thrombosis complicated by pulmonary embolism. *Journal of Neurosurgery* **560**: 179–182.
Cros D, Comp PC, Beltran G, Gum G (1990) Superior sagittal sinus thrombosis in a patient with Protein S deficiency. *Stroke* **21**: 633–636.
Cruveilhier J (1829) *Maladies du Cerveau; Inflammation des Sinus de la Dure-mere*, viiith livr. p. 4.
Curnes JT, Creasy JL, Whaley RL, Scatliff JH (1987) Air in the cavernous sinus thrombosis (Letter to the Editor). *American Journal of Neuroradiology* **8**: 176–177.
Dahlbäck B, Carlsson M, Svensson PJ (1993) Familial thrombophilia due to a previously unrecognized mechanism characterized by poor anticoagulant response to activated protein C. *Proceedings of the National Academy of Sciences (USA)* **90**: 1004.
Daif A, Awada A, Al-Rajeh S *et al.* (1995) Cerebral venous thrombosis in adults. A study of 40 cases from Saudi Arabia. *Stroke* **26**: 1193–1195.
Daniels DL, Czervionke LF, Hendrix LE *et al.* (1989) Gradient recalled echo MR imaging of superior sagittal sinus occlusion. *Neuroradiology* **31**: 134–136.
Das R, Vasishta RK, Banerjee AK (1996) Aseptic cerebral venous thrombosis associated with idiopathic ulcerative colitis: a report of two cases. *Clinical Neurology and Neurosurgery* **98:** 179–182.
David RB, Hadfield MG, Vines FS (1975) Dural sinus occlusion in leukaemia. *Pediatrics* **56**: 793–796.
Delmas MC, Cochat P, Ranchin B *et al.* (1992) Thrombose du sinus longitudinal supérieur et embolie pulmonaire au cours d'une nephrose. *Pediatrie* **47**: 31–35.
Deschiens MA, Conard J, Horrellou MH *et al.* (1996) Coagulation studies, Factor V Leiden and anticardiolipin antibodies in 40 cases of cerebral venous thrombosis. *Stroke* **27:** 1724–1730.
Deslegte RGM, Kaiser MC, Vanderbaan S, Smit L (1988) Computed tomographic diagnosis of septic sinus thrombosis and their complications. *Neuroradiology* **30**: 160–165.
Diaz JM, Schiffman JS, Urban ES, Maccario M (1992) Superior sagittal sinus thrombosis and pulmonary embolism: a syndrome rediscovered. *Acta Neurologica Scandinavica* **86**: 390–396.
Dickinson L (1896) Cases of spontaneous thrombosis of the cerebral veins and sinuses in chlorosis. *Lancet* **i**: 166.
Dindar F, Platts ME (1974) Intracranial venous thrombosis complicating oral contraception. *Canadian Medical Association Journal* **111**: 545–548.
DiNubile MJ, Boom WH, Southwick FS (1990) Septic cortical thrombophlebitis. *Journal of Infectious Diseases* **161**: 1216–1220.
DiNubile MJ (1988) Septic thrombosis of the cavernous sinuses. Neurological review. *Archives of Neurology* **45**: 567–574.
Di Rocco C, Lanelli A, Leone G *et al.* (1981) Heparin-Urokinase treatment in a septic dural sinus thrombosis. *Archives of Neurology* **38**: 431–435.
Dormont D, Anxionnat R, Evrard S *et al.* (1994) MRI in cerebral venous thrombosis. *Journal of Neuroradiology* **21**: 81–99.

Dormont D, Sag K, Biondi A *et al.* (1995) Gadolinium-enhanced MR of chronic dural sinus thrombosis. *American Journal of Neuroradiology* **16**: 1347–1352.
Dorndorf D, Wessel K, Kessler C, Kampf D (1993) Thrombosis of the right vein of Labbé: radiological and clinical findings. *Neuroradiology* **35**: 202–204.
Dowman CE (1926) Thrombosis of the Rolandic vein. *Archives of Neurology and Psychiatry* **15**: 110–112.
Doyle JB (1927) Obstruction of the longitudinal sinus. *Archives of Neurology and Psychiatry* **18**: 374–382.
Dubois J (1956) Les thrombophlébites cérébrales du post-partum. *Gynecologie et Obstétrique* **55**: 472–493.
Ducrest FM (1874) De la phlébite cérébrale et méningée chez les femmes en couches. *Archives Générales de Medicine* (4th series) **15**: 1–39.
von Dusch T (1861) *On Thrombosis of the Cerebral Sinuses*. London: The New Sydenham Society.
Dulli DA, Luzzio CC, Williams EC, Schutta HS (1996) Cerebral venous thrombosis and activated protein C resistance. *Stroke* **27**: 1431–1733.
Dunsker SB, Torres Reyes E, Peden JC (1970) Pseudotumour cerebri associated with idiopathic cryofibrinogenaemia. *Archives of Neurology* **23**: 120–127.
Duvernoy HM (1977) *Human Brainstem Vessels*. New York: Springer-Verlag.
Ecker AD (1946) Linear fracture of the skull across the venous sinuses. *New York State Journal of Medicine* **46**: 1120–1121.
Editorial (1987) Infections of the dural venous sinuses. *Lancet* **1**: 201.
Edwards MK, Kuharik MA, Cohen MD (1987). Sonographic demonstration of cerebral sinus thrombosis. *American Journal of Neuroradiology* **8**: 1153–1155.
Ehlers H, Courville CB (1936) Thrombosis of internal cerebral veins in infancy and childhood. Review of literature and report of five cases. *Journal of Pediatrics* **8**: 600–623.
Eick JJ, Miller KD, Bell KA, Tutton RH (1981) Computed tomography of deep cerebral venous thrombosis in children. *Radiology* **140**: 399–402.
Einhäupl KM, Masuhr F (1994) Cerebral venous and sinus thrombosis. An update. *European Journal of Neurology* **1**: 109–126.
Einhäupl KM, Villringer A, Haberl RL *et al.* (1990) Clinical spectrum of sinus venous thrombosis. In: *Cerebral Sinus Thrombosis: Experimental and Clinical Aspects*, Vol. 1 (eds K.M. Einhäupl, O. Kempski and A. Baethmann), pp. 149–155. New York: Plenum Press.
Einhäupl KM, Villringer A, Meister W *et al.* (1991) Heparin treatment in sinus venous thrombosis. *Lancet* **338**: 597–600.
El Koussa S, Chemaly R, Fabre Bou Abboud V *et al.* (1994) Trichinose et occlusions sino-veineuses cérébrales. *Revue Neurologique* **150**: 464–466.
Enevoldson TP, Ross Russell RW (1990) Cerebral venous thrombosis. New causes for an old syndrome. *Quarterly Journal of Medicine* **77**: 1255–1275.
Eng LJ, Longstreth WT, Shaw CM *et al.* (1990) Cerebellar venous infarction: case report with clinicopathologic correlation. *Neurology* **40**: 837–838.
Engesser L, Broekmans AW, Briet E *et al.* (1987) Hereditary protein S deficiency: clinical manifestations. *Annals of Internal Medicine* **106**: 31–36.
Eon B, Aknin P, Brun JP *et al.* (1989) Protein C deficiency and cerebral venous thrombosis in pregnancy. *Annales Francaises D'anesthesie et de Reanimation* **8**: 137–139.
Erbguth F, Brenner P, Schuierer G *et al.* (1991) Diagnosis and treatment of deep cerebral venous thrombosis. *Neurosurgical Review* **14**: 145–148.
Eskridge JM, Wessbecher FW (1991) Thrombolysis for superior sagittal sinus thrombosis. *Journal of Vascular Interventricular Radiology* **2**: 89–93.
Estanol B, Rodriguez A, Conte G *et al.* (1979) Intracranial venous thrombosis in young women. *Stroke* **10**: 680–684.
Evans RW, Patten BM (1982) Trichinosis associated with superior sagittal sinus thrombosis. *Annals of Neurology* **11**: 216–217.
Fairburn B (1973) Intracranial venous thrombosis complicating oral contraception: treatment by anticoagulant drugs. *British Medical Journal* **2**: 647.
Feldenzer JA, Bueche MJ, Venes JL, Gebarski SS (1987) Superior sagittal sinus thrombosis with infarction in sickle cell trait. *Stroke* **18**: 656–660.
Fevrier MJ, Nguyen JP, Brugieres P, Goujon C (1987) Thrombophlébite du sinus longitudinal supérieur au stade chirurgical. A propos d'un cas. Intérêt de l'Héparine de bas poids moléculaire. *Neurochirurgie* **33**: 490–493.
Finn JP, Zisk JH, Edelman RR *et al.* (1993) Central venous occlusion MR angiography. *Radiology* **187**: 245–251.

Floyd WL, Mahaley MS (1969) Cerebral venous sinus thrombosis following cardiac pacemaker implantation. *Archives of Internal Medicine* **124**: 368–372.

Foley J (1955) Benign forms of intracranial hypertension; 'toxic' and 'otitic' hydrocephalus. *Brain* **78**: 1–41.

Ford K, Sarwar M (1981) Computed tomography of dural sinus thrombosis. *American Journal of Neuroradiology* **2**: 539–543.

Freycon MT, Richard O, Allard D *et al.* (1992) Thrombose des sinus veineux intracraniens au cours d'un syndrome néphrotique. *Pediatrie* **47**: 513–516.

Fries G, Wallenfang T, Hennen J *et al.* (1992) Occlusion of the pig superior sagittal sinus, bridging and cortical veins; multi-step evolution of sinus-vein thrombosis. *Journal of Neurosurgery* **77**: 127–133.

Fujimaki T, Matsutani M, Asai A *et al.* (1986) Cerebral venous thrombosis due to high altitude polycythaemia. *Journal of Neurosurgery* **64**: 148–150.

Gabrielsen TO, Seeger JF, Knake JE, Stilwill EW (1981) Radiology of cerebral vein occlusion without dural sinus occlusion. *Radiology* **140**: 403–408.

Garcia JH (1990) Thrombosis of cranial veins and sinuses. In: *Cerebral Sinus Thrombosis* (eds K Einhäupl, O Kempski and A Baethmann) pp. 27–37. New York: Plenum Press.

Garcin R, Pestel M (1947) Sur un cas de thrombophlébite post-puerpérale. Contribution à l'étude de la pathologie veineuse de l'encéphale. *Bulletin et Memoires de la Societe Medicale des Hopitaux de Paris* **63**: 1012–1022.

Garcin R, Pestel M (1949) *Thrombo-phlébites Cérebrales.* Paris: Masson et Cie.

Gates PC (1986) Cerebral venous thrombosis: a retrospective review. *Australia and New Zealand Journal of Medicine* **16**: 766–770.

Gelle (1867) Scarlatine: phlébite des sinus de la dure-mère. *Bulletin de la Societe-Anatomique Paris,* 2nd ser. **3**: 451–453.

Gerhardt (1857) Ueber Hirnsinus – Thrombosis bei Kindern. *Deutsche Klinik* 437–438. [quoted by Kalbag and Woolf (1967)].

Gettelfinger DM, Kokmen E (1977) Superior sagittal sinus thrombosis. *Archives of Neurology* **34**: 2–6.

Go RT, Chiu CL, Neuman LA (1973) Diagnosis of superior sagittal sinus thrombosis by dynamic and sequential brain scanning. Report of one case. *Neurology* **23**: 1199–1204.

Goldberg AL, Rosenbaum AE, Wang H *et al.* (1986) Computed tomography of dural sinus thrombosis. *Journal of Computer Assisted Tomography* **10**: 16–20.

Gotoh M, Ohmoto T, Kuyama H (1993) Experimental study of venous circulatory disturbance by dural sinus occlusion. *Acta Neurochirurgica* **124**: 120–126.

Gowers WR (1893) *Manual of Diseases of the Nervous System,* Vol. 2, pp. 450–456. London: J.A. Churchill.

Graeb DA, Dolman CL (1986) Radiological and pathological aspects of dural arteriovenous fistulas. *Journal of Neurosurgery* **64**: 962–967.

Greitz T, Link H (1966) Aseptic thrombosis of intracranial sinuses. *Radiology and Clinical Biology* **35**: 111–123.

Grossman R, Novak G, Patel M *et al.* (1993) MRI in dural sinus thrombosis *Pediatric Neurology* **9:** 235–238.

Griesemer DA, Theodorou AA, Berg RA, Spera TD (1994) Local fibrinolysis in cerebral venous thrombosis. *Pediatric Neurology* **10**: 78–80.

Grove WE (1936) Septic and aseptic types of thrombosis of the cavernous sinus. *Archives of Otolaryngology* **24**: 29–50.

Guijarro C, Fernandez Carril JM, Edigo J, Gonzales JL (1995) Aseptic thrombosis of the cerebral venous sinuses and polycythaemia vera. *Neurologia* **10**: 58–59.

Haan J, Caekebeke JFV, van der Meer FJM, Wintzen AR (1988) Cerebral venous thrombosis as a presenting sign of myeloproliferative disorders. *Journal of Neurology, Neurosurgery and Psychiatry* **51**: 1219–1220.

Hacker H (1974) Normal supratentorial veins and dural sinuses. In: *Radiology of the Skull and Brain. Angiography* (eds TH Newton and DG Potts). St Louis: The C.V. Mosby Company.

Hajjar KA (1994) Factor V Leiden – an unselfish gene? *New England Journal of Medicine* **331**: 1585–1587.

Haley EC, Brasmear HR, Barth JT *et al.* (1989) Deep cerebral venous thrombosis. Clinical, neuroradiological and neuropsychological correlates. *Archives of Neurology* **46**: 337–340.

Halpern JP, Morris JGL, Driscoll GL (1984) Anticoagulants and cerebral venous thrombosis. *Australia and New Zealand Journal of Medicine* **14**: 643–648.

Hamed LM, Glaser JS, Schatz NJ, Perez FH (1989) Pseudotumor cerebri induced by Danazol. *American Journal of Ophthalmology* **107**: 105–110.

Hanigan WC, Rossi LJ, McLean JM, Wright RM (1986) MRI of cerebral vein thrombosis in infancy. A case report. *Neurology* **36**: 1354–1356.
Hanley DF, Feldman E, Borel CO *et al.* (1988) Treatment of sagittal sinus thrombosis associated with cerebral hemorrhage and intracranial hypertension. *Stroke* **19**: 903–909.
Harrison MJG, Truelove SC (1987) Cerebral venous thrombosis as a complication of ulcerative colitis. *Journal of Digestive Diseases* **12**: 1025–1028.
Hausman L (1961) *Illustrations of the Central Nervous System*. Springfield, IL: Thomas.
Hawkins DB (1985) Lateral sinus thrombosis: a sometimes unexpected diagnosis. *Laryngoscope* **95**: 674–677.
Hayes GJ (1963) External carotico-cavernous fistulas. *Journal of Neurosurgery* **20**: 692–700.
Heijer M, Blom HJ, Gerrits WBJ *et al.* (1995) Is hyperhomocysteinaemia a risk factor for recurrent venous thombosis? *Lancet* **345**: 882–885.
Heistinger M, Rumpl E, Illiasch H *et al.* (1992) Cerebral sinus thrombosis in a patient with hereditary protein S deficiency; case report and review of the literature. *Annals of Haematology* **64**: 105–109.
Hickey WF, Garnick MB, Henderson IC, Dawson DM (1982) Primary cerebral venous thrombosis in patients with cancer: a rarely diagnosed paraneoplastic syndrome. *American Journal of Medicine* **73**: 740–750.
Higashida RT, Helmer E, Halbach VV, Hieshima GB (1989) Direct thrombolytic therapy for superior sagittal sinus thrombosis. *American Journal of Neuroradiology* **10**: S4–S6.
Hillman P, Lewis SM, Bessler M *et al.* (1995) Natural history of paroxysmal nocturnal haemoglobinuria. *New England Journal of Medicine* **333**: 1253–1258.
Hirsh J, Hull R, Raskob GE (1986) Epidemiology and pathogenesis of venous thrombosis. *Journal of the American College of Cardiology* **8**: 104B–13B.
Hoch JR, Silver D (1990) Hemostasis and thrombosis. In: *Vascular Surgery*, 3rd edn (ed. WS Moore) pp. 63–79. Philadelphia: WB Saunders.
Hoffmann MW, Bill PL, Bhigjee AI *et al.* (1992) The clinicoradiological profile of cerebral venous thrombosis. *South African Medical Journal* **82**: 341–348.
Holmes G, Sargent P (1915) Injuries of the superior sagittal sinus. *British Medical Journal* **2**: 493–498.
Holt JP (1941) The collapse factor in measurement of venous pressure. *American Journal of Physiology* **134**: 292.
Horowitz M, Purdy P, Unwin H *et al.* (1995) Treatment of dural sinus thrombosis using selective catheterization and urokinase. *Annals of Neurology* **38**: 58–67.
Hosley MA, Fisher M, Lingley JF (1991) Thrombosis in a congenitally bifurcated superior sagittal sinus. *Stroke* **22**: 396–400.
Houser OW, Campbell JK, Campbell RJ, Sundt TM (1979) Arteriovenous malformation affecting the transverse dural venous sinus. An acquired lesion. *Mayo Clinic Proceedings* **54**: 651–661.
Huggenberg HR, Kesselring F (1958) Postpartum cerebral complications. *Gynaecologia* **146**: 312–317.
Hughes CE, Spear RK, Shinabarger CE, Tuna IC (1994) Septic pulmonary emboli complicating mastoiditis; Lemierre's syndrome revisited. *Clinical Infectious Diseases* **18**: 633–635.
Hughes GVR (1993) Antiphospholipid syndrome: ten years on. *Lancet* **342**: 341–344.
Huhn A (1965) Die thrombosen der intrakraniellen Venen und Sinus. Klinische und pathologisch-anatomische Untesuchungen. *Thrombosis et Diathesis Haemorrhagica* (Suppl.) 18.
Hulcelle PJ, Dooms GC, Mathurin P, Cornelis G (1989) MRI assessment of unsuspected dural sinus thrombosis. *Neuroradiology* **31**: 217–221.
Ieven M, Vael K, De Mayer M *et al.* (1993) Three cases of *Fusobacterium necrophorum* septicemia. *European Journal of Clinical Microbiology and Infectious Diseases* **12**: 705–706.
Isaacson S, Nilsson IM (1972) Defective fibrinolysis in blood and vein walls in recurrent idiopathic venous thrombosis. *Acta Chirurgica Scandinavica* **138**: 313–319.
Isensee CH, Reul J, Thron A (1994) Magnetic resonance imaging of thrombosed dural sinuses. *Stroke* **25**: 29–34.
Ivey KJ, Smith H (1968) Hypopituitarism associated with cavernous sinus thrombosis. Report of a case. *Journal of Neurology, Neurosurgery and Psychiatry* **31**: 187–189.
Jacewicz M, Plum F (1990) Aseptic cerebral venous thrombosis. In: *Cerebral Sinus Thrombosis* (eds K Einhäupl, O Kempski and A Baethmann), pp. 157–170. New York: Plenum Press.
Jackson M, Lennox G, Jaspan T, Lowe J (1993) Cerebral venous and systemic thrombosis in resolving ulcerative colitis. *Cerebrovascular Disease* **3**: 178–179.
Jaillard AS, Hommel M, Malleret M (1994) Venous sinus thrombosis associated with androgens in a healthy young man. *Stroke* **25**: 212–213.

Johnson BA, Fram EK (1992) Cerebral venous occlusive disease: pathophysiology, clinical manifestations and imaging. *Neuroimaging Clinics of North America* **2**: 769–883.

Johnson RV, Kaplan SR, Blailock ZR (1970) Cerebral venous thrombosis in paroxysmal nocturnal hemoglobinuria. *Neurology* **20**: 681–686.

Johnson S, Greenwood R, Fishman MA (1973) Internal cerebral vein thrombosis. *Archives of Neurology* **28**: 205–207.

Kalbag RM, Woolf AL (1967) *Cerebral Venous Thrombosis*, Vol. 1. London: Oxford University Press.

Kaplan B, Mickle JP (1984) In: *The Cerebral Venous System and its Disorders* (Eds JP Kapp and HH Schmidek), pp. 537–546. Orlando, FL: Grune & Stratton.

Kaplan HA (1959) The transcerebral venous system; an anatomical study. *Archives of Neurology* **1**: 148–152.

Kaplan JM, Biller J, Adams HP (1991) Outcome in non septic spontaneous superior sagittal sinus thrombosis in adults. *Cerebrovascular Disease* **1**: 231–234.

Karlin RJ, Robinson WA (1984) Septic cavernous sinus thrombosis. *Annals of Emergency Medicine* **13**: 449–455.

Keidan RD (1993) Recurrent laryngeal nerve palsy secondary to massive venous thrombosis. *Journal of Laryngology and Otology* **107**: 54–57.

Kim HS, Suzuki M, Lie JT *et al.* (1976) Clinically unsuspected disseminated intravascular coagulation. *American Journal of Clinical Pathology* **66**: 31–39.

Kim KS, Walczak TS (1986) Computed tomography of deep cerebral venous thrombosis. *Journal of Computer Assisted Tomography* **10**: 386–390.

Kimber TE, Lloyd JV, Brophy BP, Thompson PD (1996) Cerebral venous sinus thrombosis associated with factor V gene mutation *Journal of Neurology, Neurosurgery and Psychiatry* **61:** 204.

Kinal ME (1967) Traumatic thrombosis of dural venous sinuses in closed head injury. *Journal of Neurosurgery* **27**: 142–145.

Kinal ME, Jaeger RM (1960) Thrombophlebitis of dural venous sinuses following otitis media. *Journal of Neurosurgery* **17**: 81–89.

King AB (1950) Neurological conditions occurring as complications of pregnancy. *Archives of Neurology and Psychiatry* **63**: 471–499.

Kingsley DPE, Kendall BE, Moseley IF (1978) Superior sagittal sinus thrombosis, an evaluation of the changes demonstrated on computed tomography. *Journal of Neurology, Neurosurgery and Psychiatry* **41**: 1065–1068.

Komiyama A, Hirayama K, Watanabe Y (1988) Cerebral cortical vein thrombosis presenting with lobar hemorrhage in a patient with familial antithrombin III deficiency. *Clinical Neurology (Tokyo)* **298**: 493–496.

Koster T, Rosendaal FR, de Ronde H *et al.* (1993) Venous thrombosis due to poor anticoagulant response to activated protein C, Leiden thrombophilia study. *Lancet* **342**: 1503–1506.

Kozin F, Haighton V, Bernhard GC (1977) Neuro Behçet's disease; two cases and neuroradiologic findings. *Neurology* **27**: 1148–1152.

Krayenbühl H (1954) Cerebral venous thrombosis. The diagnostic value of cerebral angiogaphy. *Schweizer Archiv fuer Neurologie, Neurochirurgie und Psychiatrie* **74**: 261–287.

Krayenbühl H (1967) Cerebral venous and sinus thrombosis. *Clinical Neurosurgery* **14**: 1–24.

Krenz I, Power KJ (1990) Post partum thrombosis of the great vein of Galen. *Anaesthesia* **45**: 643–645.

Kutluk K, Schumacher M, Mironov A (1991) The role of sinus thrombosis in occipital dural arteriovenous malformations. Development and spontaneous closure. *Neurochirurgia* **34**: 144–147.

Kyritsis AP, Williams EC, Schutta HS (1990) Cerebral venous thrombosis due to heparin-induced thrombocytopenia. *Stroke* **21**: 1503–1505.

Lam BL, Schatz NJ, Glaser JS, Bowen BC (1992) Pseudotumour cerebri from cranial venous obstruction. *Ophthalmology* **99**: 706–712.

Lancereaux E (1862) *De la Thrombose et de l'Embolie Cerebrales Considerées Principalement dans leur Rapport avec le Ramollissement du Cerveau*. Paris: Adrien Delahaye Libraire.

Lang J, Schneider W (1989) The superficial cerebral veins. *Gegenbaurs Morphologisches Jahrbuch* **135**: 271–303.

Lavin PJM, Bone J (1978) Intracranial venous thrombosis in the first trimester of pregnancy. *Journal of Neurology, Neurosurgery and Psychiatry* **41**: 726–729.

Lau SU, Bock GH, Edson JR, Michael AF (1980) Sagittal sinus thrombosis in the nephrotic syndrome. *Journal of Pediatrics* **97**: 948–950.

Laversuch CJ, Brown MM, Clifton A, Bourke BE (1995) Cerebral venous thrombosis and acquired protein S deficiency: an uncommon cause of headache in systemic lupus erythematosus. *British Journal of Rheumatology* **34:** 572–575.

Leslie ML, Stein RL, Galloway P (1987) Cerebral thrombosis in patients with systemic lupus erythematosus. *Journal of Neurology, Neurosurgery and Psychiatry* **50**: 1701–1702.

Levine SR, Puziok KS, Feith Patel, SG, Welch KMA (1987) Cerebral venous thrombosis with lupus anticoagulant – Report of 2 cases. *Stroke* **18**: 801–804.

Levine SR, Twyman RE, Gilman S (1988) The role of anticoagulation in cavernous sinus thrombosis. *Neurology* **38**: 517–521.

Levine SR, Deegan MJ, Futrell N, Welch KMA (1990) Cerebrovascular and neurologic disease associated with antiphospholipid antibodies. *Neurology* **40**: 1181–1189.

Lidell JA (1874) On thrombosis of the cerebral veins and sinuses of the dura mater. *American Journal of Medical Sciences* (NS) **67**: 39–65.

Lyman R (1935) The pros and cons of jugular vein ligation for lateral sinus thrombosis. *Kentucky Medical Journal* **33**: 351–354.

Macchi PJ, Grossman RI, Gomori JM *et al.* (1986) High field MR imaging of cerebral venous thrombosis. *Journal of Computer Assisted Tomography* **10**: 10–15.

Martin JP (1944) Venous thrombosis in the central nervous system. *Proceedings of the Royal Society of Medicine* **37**: 383–386.

Martin JP (1955) Signs of obstruction of the superior longitudinal sinus following closed head injuries (traumatic hydrocephalus). *British Medical Journal* **ii**: 467–470.

Martin JP, Sheehan HL (1941) Primary thrombosis of cerebral veins (following childbirth). *British Medical Journal* **1**: 349–353.

Martinelli I, Land G, Merati G, Cella R, Tosetto A, Munucci PM (1996) Factor V gene mutation is a risk factor for cerebral venous thrombosis. *Thrombosis and Haemostasis* **75**: 393–394.

Mas JL, Meder JF, Meary E, Bousser MG (1990) Magnetic resonance imaging in lateral sinus hypoplasia and thrombosis. *Stroke* **21**: 1350–1356.

Mas JL, Meder JF, Meary E (1992) Dural sinus thrombosis: long-term follow up by magnetic resonance imaging. *Cerebrovascular Disease* **2**: 137–144.

Masheter HC (1959) Behçet's syndrome complicated by intracranial thrombophlebitis. *Proceedings of the Royal Society of Medicine* **52**: 1039–1040.

Matthew NT, Abraham J, Taori GM, lyer GV (1971). Inernal carotid artery occlusion in cavernous sinus thrombosis. *Archives of Neurology* **24**: 11–16.

Mattle H, Edelman RR, Reis MA, Atkinson DJ (1990) Flow quantification in the superior sagittal sinus using magnetic resonance. *Neurology* **40**: 813–815.

Mattle HP, Wentz KU, Edelman RR *et al.* (1991) Cerebral venography with MR. *Radiology* **178**: 453–458.

McArdle CB, Mirfakhraee M, Amparo EG, Kulkarni MV (1987) MR imaging of transverse/sigmoid dural sinus and jugular vein thrombosis. *Journal of Computer Assisted Tomography* **11**: 831–838.

McCulloch J, Edvinson L, Watts P (1982) Comparison of the effects of K and pH on the calibre of cerebral veins and arteries. *Pfluger's Archives* **393**: 95–98.

McMurdo SK, Brant-Zawadzki M, Bradley WG *et al.* (1986) Dural sinus thrombosis study using intermediate field strength MR imaging. *Radiology* **161**: 83–86.

Medlock MD, Olivero WC, Hanigan WC *et al.* (1992) Children with cerebral venous thrombosis diagnosed with magnetic resonance imaging and magnetic resonance angiography. *Neurosurgery* **31**: 870–876.

Meininger V, James JM, Rio B, Zittoun R (1985) Occlusions des sinus veineux de la dure-mère au cours des hémopathies. *Revue Neurologique* **141**: 228–233.

Melamed E, Rachmilewicz EA, Reches A, Lavy S (1976) Aseptic cavernous sinus thrombosis after internal carotid artery occlusion in polycythaemia vera. *Journal of Neurology, Neurosurgery and Psychiatry* **39**: 320–324.

Merwarth HR (1942) The syndrome of the Rolandic vein. *American Journal of Surgery* **56**: 526–544.

Meyohas M-C, Roullet E, Rouzioux C *et al.* (1989) Cerebral venous thrombosis and dural primary infection with HIV and cytomegalovirus. *Journal of Neurology, Neurosurgery and Psychiatry* **52**: 1010–1011.

Micheli F, Schteinschnaider A, Plaghos LL *et al.* (1989) Bacterial cavernous sinus aneurysm treated by detachable balloon technique. *Stroke* **20**: 1751–1754.

Mickle JP, McLennan JE, Chi JG, Lidden CW (1977) Cortical vein thrombosis in Wegener's granulomatosis. *Journal of Neurosurgery* **46**: 248–251.

Milandre L, Gueriot C, Girard N *et al.* (1988) Les thromboses veineuses cérébrales de l'adulte. *Annales de Medécine Interne* **139**: 544–554.

Mills JL, Taylor LM, Porter JM (1987) Buerger's disease in the modern era. *American Journal of Surgery* **154**: 123–129.

Mineta T, Fukuyama K, Matsumoto S, Kishikawa T, Tabuchi K (1991) Dural arterio-venous malformation associated with occlusion of the superior sagittal sinus – a case report. *Neurologia Medico-Chirurgica* **31:** 41–44.
Miyata T, Yamada N, Iida Y *et al.* (1994) Abnormalities of PIG-A transcripts in granulocytes from patients with paroxysmal nocturnal hemoglobinuria. *New England Journal of Medicine* **330**: 249–255.
Mohamed A, McLeod JG, Hallinan J (1991) Superior sagittal sinus thrombosis. *Clinical and Experimental Neurology* **28**: 23–36.
Mones RJ (1965) Increased intracranial pressure due to metastatic disease of venous sinuses. *Neurology* **15**: 1000–1007.
Montrieul B, Janny P (1962) Contribution à l'étude angiographique des thromboses veineuses cérébrales. *Neurochirurgie* **8**: 175–188.
Montalban J, Codina A, Ordi J *et al.* (1991) Antiphospholipid antibodies in cerebral ischaemia. *Stroke* **22**: 751–753.
Moorhead JG, Abramson L (1928) Thrombophlebitis migrans. *British Medical Journal* **i**: 586–587.
Morvas S, Morvas I (1968) Carotid-cavernous fistula complicating cavernous sinus thrombophlebitis. *Clinical Radiology* **19**: 91–94.
Motte S, Flamme F, Depianeux M, Wantrecht JC *et al.* (1992) Venous thromboangiitis associated with regional enteritis. *Internal Angiology* **11**: 237–240.
Muir KW (1995) Anticardiolipin antibodies and cardiovascular diseases. *Journal of the Royal Society of Medicine* **88**: 433–436.
Murphy MF, Clarke CRA, Brearley RL (1983) Superior sagittal sinus thrombosis and essential thrombocythaemia. *British Medical Journal* **287**: 1344.
Nagpal RD (1983) Dural sinus and cerebral venous thrombosis. *Neurosurgical Review* **6**: 155–160.
Nakahara I, Pile-Spellman J, Hacein-Bey L *et al.* (1993) Posterior fossa dural arterio-venous fistula with isolated sinus segment. *Brain and Nerve* **45**: 703–709.
Nayak AK, Karnad D, Mahajan MV *et al.* (1994) Cerebellar venous infarction in chronic suppurative otitis media. A case report with review of four other cases. *Stroke* **25**: 1958–1960.
Newman DS, Levine SR, Curtis VL, Welch KMA (1989) Migraine-like visual phenomena associated with cerebral venous thrombosis. *Headache* **29**: 82–85.
Newton TH, Hoyt WF (1970) Dural arterio-venous shunts in the region of the cavernous sinus. *Neuroradiology* **1**: 71–81.
Nishimura RN, Stepanek D, Howieson J, Hammerstad J (1982) Internal cerebral vein thrombosis. A case report. *Archives of Neurology* **39**: 439–440.
Noetzel H, Jerusalem F (1965) Die Hirnvenen und sinusthrombosen. *Monographien aus dem Gesamtgebiete der Neurologie und Psychiatrie* **106**: 1–63.
O'Connell JE (1990) Lateral sinus thrombosis. A problem still with us. *Journal of Laryngology and Otology* **104**: 949–951.
Odake G (1992) Meningioma of the falco-tentorial region: report of two cases. *Neurosurgery* **30**: 788–793.
Oguz M, Aksungur EH, Soyupak SH, Yildirum AU (1994) Vein of Galen and sinus thrombosis with bilateral thalamic infarcts in sickle cell anaemia. *Neuroradiology* **36**: 155–156.
Osborn AG, Anderson RE, Wing SD (1980) The false falx sign. Radiology **134**: 421–425.
Padayachee TS, Bingham JB, Graves MJ *et al.* (1991) Dural sinus thrombosis. Diagnosis and follow-up by magnetic resonance angiography and imaging. *Neuroradiology* **33**: 165–167.
Pamir MN, Kansu T, Erbengi A, Zileli (1981) Papilledema in Behçet syndrome. *Archives of Neurology* **38**: 643–645.
Parrot MJ (1873) Etude sur les ramollissements de l'encéphale chez le nouveau-né. *Archives de Physiologie Normale et Pathologique* **5**: 59–73.
Pasquale LR, Moster ML, Schmaier A (1990) Dural sinus thrombosis with abnormalities of protein S and fibrinogen. *Archives of Ophthalmology* **108**: 644.
Patchell RA, Posner JB (1986) Neurologic complications of carcinoid. *Neurology* **36**: 745–749.
Patronas NJ, Duda EE, Mirfakhraee M, Wollmann RL (1981) Superior sagittal sinus thrombosis diagnosed by computed tomography. *Surgical Neurology* **15**: 11–14.
Pennybacker J, (1943) Papilloedema due to intracranial venous obstruction. *Transactions of the Ophthalmology Society of the UK*, 333–338.
Perese BM (1960) Superficial veins of the brain from a surgical point of view. *Journal of Neurosurgery* **17**: 402–412.
Persson L, Lilja A (1990) Extensive dural sinus thrombosis treated by surgical removal and local streptokinase infusion. *Neurosurgery* **26**: 117–121.

Phillips G (1948) Cerebral thrombophlebitis and fibrinogen B. *Journal of Neurology, Neurosurgery and Psychiatry* **11**: 236.

Plant GT, Donald JJ, Jackowski A *et al.* (1991) Partial non-thrombotic superior sagittal sinus occlusion due to occipital skull tumours. *Journal of Neurology, Neurosurgery and Psychiatry* **54**: 520–523.

Poltera AA (1972) The pathology of intracranial venous thrombosis in oral contraception. *Journal of Pathology* **106**: 209–219.

Preter M, Tzourio Ch, Ameri A, Bousser MG (1996) Long term prognosis in cerebral venous thrombosis. A follow up of 77 patients. *Stroke* **27**: 243–246.

Rao KCVG, Knipp HC, Wagner EJ (1981) CT findings in cerebral sinus and venous thrombosis. *Radiology* **140**: 391–398.

Raveh E, Cohen M, Shpitzer T, Feinmesser R (1995) Carcinoma of the thyroid: a cause of hypercoagulability? *Ear Nose and Throat Journal* **74**: 110–112.

Ray BS, Dunbar HS (1951) Thrombosis of dural venous sinuses as cause of 'pseudotumor cerebri'. *Annals of Surgery* **134**: 376–386.

Reading PV, Schurr P (1956) Thrombosis of the sigmoid sinus. *Lancet* **2**: 473–476.

Ribes F (1825) Des reserches faites sur la phlébite. *Revue de Médicine* **3**: 5.

Rich C, Gill JC, Wernick S, Konkol KJ (1993) An unusual case of cerebral venous thrombosis in a child. *Stroke* **24**: 603–605.

Rippe DJ, Boyko OB, Spritzer CE *et al.* (1990) Demonstration of dural sinus occlusion by the use of MR angiography. *American Journal of Neuroradiology* **11**: 199–201.

Rivkin MJ, Anderson ML, Kaye EM (1992) Neonatal idiopathic cerebral venous thrombosis: an unrecognized cause of transient seizures or lethargy. *Annals of Neurology* **32**: 51–56.

Rondepierre Ph, Hamon M, Leys D *et al.* (1995) Thromboses veineuses cérébrales: étude de l'évolution. *Revue Neurologique* **151**: 100–104.

Ross J (1881) *A Treatise on Diseases of the Nervous System*, Vol. 2, 1st edn, pp. 518–523. London.

Ross WF (1982) Treatment of paroxysmal nocturnal hemoglobinuria. *Blood* **60**: 20–23.

Ross Russell RW (1966) A study of the microcirculation in experimental cerebral embolism. *Angiologica* **3**: 240–258.

Rothwell M, Grant R (1993) Cerebral venous sinus thrombosis induced by ecstasy. *Journal of Neurology, Neurosurgery and Psychiatry* **56**: 1035.

Rousseaux P, Bernard MH, Scherpereel B, Guyot JF (1978) Thrombose des sinus veineux intracrâniens (à propos de 22 cas). *Neurochirurgie* **24**: 197–203.

Rousseaux M, Lesoin F, Barbaste P, Jomin M (1988) Infarctus cérébelleux pseudo-tumoral d'origine veineuse. *Revue Neurologique* **144**: 209–211.

Ruel M, Montfort JC, Pinta P (1986) Symptomatologie trompeuse des thrombophlébites cérébrales au cours de la grossesse et du post-partum. *Presse Medicale* **15**: 1367–1368.

Rüttner HB (1991) Die aseptische zerebrale sinusthrombose. *Schweisenische Medizinische Wochenschrift* **121**: 1601–1611.

Sakurai N, Koike Y, Hashizume Y, Takahashi A (1992) Dural arteriovenous malformation and sinus thrombosis in a patient with prostatic cancer; an autopsy case. *Internal Medicine* **31**: 1032–1037.

Samama M, Horellou MH, Soria J *et al.* (1984) Successful progressive anticoagulation in a severe protein C deficiency and previous skin necrosis at the initiation of oral anticoagulant treatment. *Thrombosis and Haemostasis* **51**: 132–133.

Samuel J, Fernandes CM (1987) Lateral sinus thrombosis. A review of 45 cases. *Journal of Laryngology and Otology* **101**: 1227–1229.

Saponaro SA, Flanders AE, Friedman DP, Mandel S (1994) Superior sagittal sinus thrombosis in the presence of idiopathic bilateral internal jugular vein thrombosis. *Journal of Neuroimaging* **4**: 48–50.

Sauron B, Chiras J, Chain F, Castaigne P (1982) Thrombophlébite cérébelleuse chez un homme porteur d'un déficit familial en antithromboine III. *Revue Neurologique* **138**: 685.

Savino PJ, Grossman RI, Schatz NJ *et al.* (1986) High field magnetic resonance imaging in the diagnosis of cavernous sinus thrombosis. *Archives of Neurology* **43**: 1081–1082.

Schafer AI (1984) Bleeding and thrombosis in the myeloproliferative disorders. *Blood* **64**: 1–12.

Schenk EA (1964) Sickle cell trait and superior sagittal sinus thrombosis. *Annals of Internal Medicine* **60**: 465–470.

Schutta HS, Williams EC, Baranski BG, Sutula TP (1991) Cerebral venous thrombosis with plasminogen deficiency. *Stroke* **22**: 401–405.

Scott JA, Pascuzzi RM, Hall PV, Becker GJ (1988) Treatment of dural sinus thrombosis with local urokinase infusion. *Journal of Neurosurgery* **68**: 284–287.

Segall HD, Ahmadi J, McComb JG *et al.* (1982) Computed tomographic observations pertinent to intracranial venous thrombotic and occlusive disease in childhood. *Radiology* **143**: 441–449.
Sekhar LN, Dujouny M, Rao GR (1980) Carotid cavernous sinus thrombosis caused by aspergillus fumigatus. *Journal of Neurosurgery* **52**: 120–125.
Shaw RE (1952) Cavernous sinus thrombosis: a review. *British Journal of Surgery* **40**: 40–48.
Shevell MI, Silver K, O'Gorman AM, Watters GV, Montes JL (1989) Neonatal dural sinus thrombosis. *Pediatric Neurology* **15**: 161–165.
Shinohara Y, Yosmitoshi M, Yoshii F (1986) Appearance and disappearance of empty delta sign in superior sagittal sinus thrombosis. *Stroke* **17**: 1282–1284.
Shiozawa Z, Yamada H, Mabuchi C *et al.* (1982) Superior sagittal sinus thrombosis associated with androgen therapy for hypoplastic anaemia. *Annals of Neurology* **12**: 578–580.
Sigsbee B, Rotenberg DA (1978) Sagittal sinus thrombosis as a complication of regional enteritis. *Annals of Neurology* **3**: 450–452.
Sigsbee B, Deck MDF, Posner JB (1979) Non-metastatic superior sagittal sinus thrombosis complicating systemic cancer. *Neurology* **29**: 139–146.
Silburn PA, Sandstrom PA, Staples C *et al.* (1996) Deep cerebral venous thrombosis presenting as an encephalitic illness. *Postgraduate Medical Journal* **72:** 355–357.
Silverstein A, Gilbert H, Wasserman LR (1962) Neurologic complications of polycythemia. *Annals of Internal Medicine* **57**: 909–916.
Sindou M, Mercier P, Brunon J *et al.* (1980) Hypertension intra-crânienne 'bénigne' par thrombose des deux sinus latéraux traitée par pontage veineux. *Nouvelle Presse Medicale* **9**: 439–442.
Singh B (1993) The management of lateral sinus thrombosis. *Journal of Laryngology and Otology* **107**: 803–808.
Sjolin S (1959) Studies in osteopetrosis. *Acta Paediatrica Scandinavica* **48**: 532–546.
Smith BH (1984) Infections of the dura and its venous sinuses. In: *Clinical Neurology*, Vol. 2 (eds AB Baker and LH Baker), pp. 28. Philadelphia: Harper and Row.
Smith TP, Higashida R, Barnwell S *et al.* (1994) Treatment of dural sinus thrombosis by urokinase infusion. *AJNR* **15**: 801–807.
Smith WDF, Sinar J, Carey M (1983) Sagittal sinus thrombosis and occult malignancy. *Journal of Neurology, Neurosurgery and Psychiatry* **46**: 187–188.
Snyder TC, Sachdev HS (1986) MR imaging of cerebral dural sinus thrombosis. *Journal of Computer Assisted Tomography* **10**: 889–891.
Solomon GE, Engel M, Hecht HL, Rapoport AR (1982) Progressive dyskinesia due to internal cerebral vein thrombosis. *Neurology* **32**: 769–772.
Souter RG, Mitchell A (1982) Spreading cortical venous thrombosis due to infusion of hyperosmolar solutions into the internal jugular vein. *British Medical Journal* **285**: 935–936.
Southwick FS, Richardson EP Jr, Swartz MN (1986) Septic thrombosis of the dural venous sinuses. *Medicine* **65**: 82–106.
Srinivasan K (1983) Cerebral venous and arterial thrombosis in pregnancy and puerperium. *Angiology* **34**: 731–746.
Stam J (1993) Treatment of cerebral venous thrombosis. *Cerebrovascular Disease* **3**: 329–330.
Stam J, Lensing AWA, Vermeulen M, Tijssen JGP (1991) Heparin treatment for cerebral venous and sinus thrombosis. *Lancet* **338**: 1154.
Stansfield FR (1942) Puerperal cerebral thrombophlebitis treated by heparin. *British Medical Journal* **1**: 436–438.
Stehle G, Buss J, Heene DL (1991) Non infectious thrombosis of the superior sagittal sinus in a patient with iron deficiency anaemia. *Stroke* **22**: 414.
Steinherz PG, Miller LP, Ghavimi F *et al.* (1981) Dural sinus thrombosis in children with acute lymphoblastic leukaemia. *Journal of the American Medical Association* **246**: 2837–2839.
Stephens PH, Lennox G, Hirsch N, Miller D (1991) Superior sagittal sinus thrombosis after internal jugular vein cannulation. *British Journal of Anaesthesia* **67**: 476–479.
Stevens H, Ammerman HH (1959) Intracranial venous thrombosis in early pregnancy. *American Journal of Obstetrics and Gynecology* **78**: 104–108.
Svensson PJ, Dahlbäck B (1994) Resistance to activated protein C as a basis for venous thrombosis. *New England Journal of Medicine* **330**: 517–522.
Swanson HS, Fincher EF (1954) Experience involving superior longitudinal sinus and rolandic veins. *Neurology* **4**: 801–810.
Symonds CP (1937) Hydrocephalic and focal cerebral symptoms in relation to thrombophlebitis of the dural sinuses and cerebral veins. *Brain* **60**: 531–550.

Symonds CP (1940) Cerebral thrombophlebitis. *British Medical Journal* **2**: 348–352.
Symonds CP (1944) Venous thrombosis in the central nervous system (discussion). *Proceedings of the Royal Society of Medicine* **37**: 386–387.
Symonds CP (1956) Otitic hydrocephalus. *Neurology* **6**: 681–685.
Sze G, Simmons B, Krol G *et al.* (1988) Dural sinus thrombosis: verification with spin echo techniques. *American Journal of Neuroradiology* **9**: 679–686.
Tajima Y, Minami N, Okumura K *et al.* (1991) An unusual case of superior sagittal sinus thrombosis with dural AV fistula. *No to Shinkei – Brain and Nerve* **43**: 981–985.
Tarras S, Gadia C, Mester L *et al.* (1988) Homozygous protein C deficiency in a newborn. Clinicopathologic correlation. *Archives of Neurology* **45**: 214–220.
Taylor GA (1992) Intracranial venous system in the newborn. Evaluation of normal anatomy and flow characteristics with color Döppler ultrasound. *Radiology* **183**: 449–452.
Tehindrazanarivelo AD, Bousser MG (1994) Idiopathic intracranial hypertension and cerebral dural sinus thrombosis. *American Journal of Medicine* **97**: 200–201.
Tehindrazanarivelo AD, Evrard S, Schaison M *et al.* (1992) Prospective study of cerebral sinus venous thrombosis in patients presenting with benign intracranial hypertension. *Cerebrovascular Disease* **2**: 22–27.
Tezzon F, Ferrari G, Sbarbaro V, *et al.* (1994) Deep cerebral venous thrombosis and hereditary tissue plasminogen activator(tPA) deficiency. *Italian Journal of Neurological Sciences* **15:** 507–512.
Thron A, Wessel K, Linden D, Schroth G, Dichgans A (1986) Superior sagittal sinus thrombosis: neuroradiological evaluation and clinical findings. *Journal of Neuroradiology* **233**: 283.
Toglia MR, Weg JG (1996) Venous thrombosis during pregnancy. *New England Journal of Medicine* **335**: 108–114.
Tonnelle M-L (1829) Memoire sur les maladies des sinus veineux de la dure-mère. *Journal Hebdomadaire de Médecine* **5**: 337–403.
Tovi F, Fliss DM, Noyek AM (1993) Septic internal jugular vein thrombosis. *Journal of Otolaryngology* **22**: 415–420.
Towbin A (1973) The syndrome of latent cerebral venous thrombosis; its frequency and relation to age and congestive heart failure. *Stroke* **4**: 419–430.
Tsai FY, Higashida RT, Matovich V, Alfieri K (1992) Acute thrombosis of the intracranial dural sinus: direct thrombolytic treatment. *American Journal of Neuroradiology* **13**: 1137–1141.
Tsai FY, Wang AM, Matovich VB *et al.* (1995) MR staging of acute dural sinus thrombosis: correlation with venous pressure measurements and implications for treatment and prognosis. *American Journal of Neuroradiology* **16**: 1021–1029.
Tsuruda JS, Shimakawa A, Pecl NJ, Saloner D (1991) Dural sinus occlusions. Evaluation with phase sensitive gradient echo MR imaging. *American Journal of Neuroradiology* **12**: 481–488.
Urban E, Jabbari B, Robles H (1994) Concurrent cerebral venous sinus thrombosis and myeloradiculopathy in Sjögren's syndrome. *Neurology* **44**: 554–556.
Ur Rahman N, Al-Tahan AR (1993) Computed tomographic evidence of an extensive thrombosis and infarction of the deep venous system. *Stroke* **24**: 744–746.
Vaezi MF, Rustagi PK, Elson CO (1995) Transient protein S deficiency associated with cerebral venous thrombosis in active ulcerative colitis. *American Journal of Gastroenterology* **90:** 313–315.
Valdueza JM, Schultz M, Harms L, Einhäupl KM (1995) Venous transcranial Döppler ultrasound monitoring in acute dural sinus thrombosis. Report of two cases. *Stroke* **26**: 1196–1199.
Van Dyke DC, Eldadah MK, Bale JF Jr *et al.* (1992) Mycoplasma pneumoniae-induced cerebral venous thrombosis treated with urokinase. *Clinical Pediatrics* **31**: 501–504.
Van Vleymen B, Dehaene I, van Hoof A, Pattyn G (1987) Cerebral venous thrombosis in paroxysmal nocturnal haemoglobinuria. *Acta Neurologica Belgica* **87**: 80–87.
Vernant JC, Delaporte, JM, Buisson G *et al.* (1988) Cerebrovascular complications of sickle cell anaemia. *Revue Neurologique* **144**: 465–473.
Vidailhet M, Piette JC, Wechsler B *et al.* (1990) Cerebral venous thrombosis in systemic lupus erythematosus. *Stroke* **21**: 1226–1231.
Vieregge P, Schweider G, Kompf D (1989) Cerebral venous thrombosis in hereditary protein C deficiency. *Journal of Neurology, Neurosurgery and Psychiatry* **52**: 135–137.
Villringer A, Seiderer M, Bauer WM *et al.* (1989) Diagnosis of superior sagittal sinus thrombosis by three-dimensional magnetic resonance flow imaging. *Lancet* **i**: 1086–1087.
Villringer A, Bousser MG, Einhäupl KM (1994) Cerebral sinus venous thrombosis. In: *Neurocritical Care*, Vol. 1 (ed. W. Hacke), pp. 654–660. Berlin: Springer Verlag.
Villringer A, Mehraein S, Einhäupl KM (1994a) Pathophysiological aspects of cerebral sinus venous thrombosis (CSVT). *Journal of Neuroradiology* **21**: 72–80.

Villringer A, Mehraein S, Einhäupl KM (1994b) Treatment of sinus venous thrombosis – beyond the recommendation of anticoagulation. *Journal of Neuroradiology* **21**: 72–80.

Vines FS, Davis DO (1971) Clinical–radiological correlation in cerebral venous occlusive disease. *Radiology* **98**: 9–22.

Virapongse C, Cazenave C, Quisling R *et al.* (1987) The empty delta sign: frequency and significance in 76 cases of dural sinus thrombosis. *Radiology* **162**: 779–785.

Vogl TJ, Balzer JO, Stemmler J *et al.* (1992) MR angiography in children with cerebral neurovascular diseases: findings in 31 cases. *American Journal of Roentgenology* **159**: 817–823.

Vogl TJ, Bergman C, Villringer A *et al.* (1994) Dural sinus thrombosis: value of venous MR angiography for diagnosis and follow-up. *American Journal of Roentgenology* **162**: 1191–1198.

Waddington MM (1974) *Atlas of Cerebral Angiography with Anatomic Correlation*. Boston: Little Brown and Company.

Waggoner RW (1928) Thrombosis of a superior cerebral vein. *Archives of Neurology and Psychiatry* **20**: 580–584.

Wardlaw JM, Vaughan GT, Steers AJW, Sellar RJ (1994) Transcranial Döppler ultrasound findings in venous sinus thrombosis. *Journal of Neurosurgery* **80**: 332–335.

Wechsler B, Vidailhet M, Piette JC *et al.* (1992) Cerebral venous thrombosis in Behçet's disease: clinical study and long-term follow-up of 25 cases. *Neurology* **42**: 614–618.

Weesner CL, Cisek JE (1993) Lemierre's syndrome; the forgotten disease. *Annals of Emergency Medicine* **22**: 256–258.

Weinmann EE, Salzman EW (1994) Deep vein thrombosis. *New England Journal of Medicine* **331**: 1630–1641.

Weisman AD (1944) Cavernous sinus thrombophlebitis: report of a case with multiple cerebral infarcts and necrosis of pituitary body. *New England Journal of Medicine* **231**: 118–120.

Williams RS, Richardson EP (1988) Case records of the Massachussetts General Hospital. *New England Journal of Medicine* **318**: 1322–1328.

Wintzen AR, Broekmans AW, Bertina RM *et al.* (1985) Cerebral haemorrhagic infarcts in young patients with hereditary protein C deficiency. *British Medical Journal* **290**: 350–352.

Woodhall B (1936) Variations of the cranial venous sinuses in the region of the torcular herophili. *Archives of Surgery* **33**: 297–310.

Yarrington CT (1977) Cavernous sinus thrombosis revisited. *Proceedings of the Royal Society of Medicine* **70**: 456–459.

Yasargil MG, Damur M (1974) Thrombosis of the cerebral veins and dural sinuses. In: *Radiology of the Skull and Brain. Angiography* (eds TH Newton and DG Potts). St Louis: The C.V. Mosby Company.

Yerby MS, Bailey GM (1980) Superior sagittal sinus thrombosis ten years after surgery for ulcerative colitis. *Stroke* **11**: 294–296.

Yokota T, Ishiai S, Furukawa T, Tsukagoshi H (1990) Pure agraphia of kanji due to thrombosis of the Labbé vein. *Journal of Neurology, Neurosurgery and Psychiatry* **53**: 335–338.

Yokota M, Tani E, Maeda Y, Yamaura I (1993) Meningioma in the sigmoid sinus groove associated with dural arteriovenous malformation. *Neurosurgery* **33**: 316–319.

Yoshii N, Seiki Y, Samejima H *et al.* (1978) Occlusion of the deep cerebral veins. *Neuroradiology* **16**: 287–288.

Yuh WT, Simonson TM, Wang AM *et al.* (1994) Venous sinus occlusive disease: MR findings. *American Journal of Neuroradiology* **15**: 309–316.

Zuber M, Toulon P, Marnet L, Mas JL (1996) Factor V Leiden mutation in cerebral venous thrombosis *Stroke* **27**: 1721–1723.

Index